Praise f

Tufton's firsthand experience provides a riveting and inspiring narrative of crisis management in *Wild Flavours*. His detailed account offers a unique perspective on leadership during the pandemic.

Dr. Aaron Poynton | CEO, Omnipoynt Solutions and *USA Today and WSJ* Best-selling Author

Wild Flavours reads more like a masterly paced thriller than a political memoir. Chris Tufton's electrifyingly candid account of COVID-19 gives readers a rare ringside seat at the heart of one island's battle against a global pandemic. Gripping, humane, vividly personal and endlessly revelatory, I couldn't put it down. Jamaica's good fortune to have a Minister of Health equal to the crisis is now all of ours. Before reading his book, I thought I already knew the story of COVID-19. This masterclass in storytelling proves not just how wrong I was, but that even from a worldwide catastrophe, something beautiful can come.

Decca Aitkenhead | Chief Interviewer, *Sunday Times*

Chris Tufton's *Wild Flavours* is an inspiring and meticulously detailed account of Jamaica's response to the COVID-19 pandemic. As a healthcare leader myself, I am particularly impressed by Tufton's emphasis on transparency, trust, and decisive action—values that resonate deeply with my own experiences during the pandemic.

The book is a testament to the power of leadership in a crisis, vividly portraying how decisive leadership, clear communication, and collective action can guide a nation through unprecedented challenges. Tufton's narrative is a valuable resource for leaders across all sectors, showcasing the importance of unity and openness in navigating a public health crisis.

Dr. Sandra Lindsay | Northwell Health's Vice President of Public Health Advocacy

Wild Flavours is a comprehensive and compelling account of Jamaica's fight against COVID-19. It is rich with lessons for future leaders, with the narrative offering deep insights into crisis leadership and response.

Casel Burnett | International Best-selling Author

Wild Flavours provides a detailed and painstaking account of a public health crisis from the view of a main actor, Chris Tufton, Minister of Health and Wellness. The book covers diverse topics such as the arrival of patient zero to geopolitics and vaccination. It has rich empirical data on the anatomy of the crisis in Jamaica spread across fifty-six sections. It is a fascinating read and should be made compulsory reading for public health leaders.

Densil A. Williams | Professor of International Business, Pro Vice Chancellor and Principal, University of the West Indies, Mona

Wild Flavours tells Jamaica's tale in the way only Dr. the Honorable Christopher Tufton can—with candor, calmly but so captivatingly that you don't want to put this book down. He is true to the Jamaican culture and stark in his descriptions of the never-ending struggles that faced Jamaica's health system. The thing I appreciate is that he captures the secret of Caribbean pride—struggle does not mean surrender. In the Caribbean, once there is life—there is hope.

Dr. Joy St. John | Executive Director, Caribbean Public Health Agency

Dr. Chris Tufton has written a must-read account of Jamaica's turbulent yet successful navigation of the COVID-19 pandemic, which will serve as a reference tool for years to come.

Sharon J. Miller | Ambassador, Jamaica

Behind the scenes of the worst health catastrophe the world has experienced in a century, *Wild Flavours* showcases the bravery and resilience of Jamaica's frontline workers. This book illuminates the challenges and sacrifices made during the pandemic, making it a must-read for anyone interested in public health and crisis response.

Maria Claudia Hoepers | Entrepreneur and Best-Selling Author

WILD FLAVOURS

An Insider Account of Jamaica's Journey
Through the Crisis of the COVID-19 Pandemic

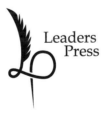

Leaders
Press

CHRIS TUFTON

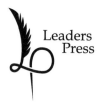

ISBN 978-1-63735-329-5 (pbk)
ISBN 978-1-63735-330-1 (hcv)
ISBN 978-1-63735-328-8 (ebook)

Library of Congress Control Number: 2024914896

Table of Contents

To Jamaica's frontline public health workers, especially those who died serving their country, protecting Jamaicans from illness

Prologue: Patient Zero |

When Patient Zero stepped off the British Airways flight from London to Kingston on Wednesday, March 4, 2020, she had no idea that she would be the first COVID-19 case in Jamaica. She had traveled with her husband and their two-year-old son to attend a family funeral. Her aunt, who she considered her granny, had passed away. This was a final send-off she could not miss.

Happy to be home for the first time in several years, Patient Zero— the epidemiological team later re-designated her Patient One— visited with friends and family in Seven Mile, Bull Bay, a semi-rural community on Kingston's eastern outskirts. This was the first time they were meeting her son, a source of happiness for everyone.

She stayed in Seven Mile, at a large extended family compound containing several households where seventy-four people lived. Across the road lived other family members, and she moved back and forth between the two premises throughout the day.

She visited her father in Mocho, Clarendon, in the centre of the island heading west. It was a ninety-minute drive; she had an arrangement with a trusted taxi driver from the nearby community of Wickie Wackie, who had picked her up from the airport, and provided her transportation for her stay in Jamaica. He was a careful driver. His car was reliable, and it had air conditioning. She visited the Rest Haven Funeral Home, just a mile or so up the road, as she got involved in the funeral preparations. A wake was scheduled on Friday, the first of several family gatherings centred on granny's passing. The funeral was on Saturday, at the Grace Gospel Hall in Harbour View. The burial followed at the Meadowrest Memorial Garden in St. Catherine.

On Sunday, March 8, Patient One began to feel unwell—feverish, with a slight cough. The following Monday morning, she felt worse. At no time did she consider she had the novel coronavirus. While it was spreading in England, especially in London, she had not known anyone who had been afflicted.

A family member took her to a doctor, who quickly recognized her symptoms as the coronavirus, and she was immediately transferred to the University Hospital of the West Indies (UHWI), where she was put in isolation. The Ministry of Health and Wellness (MOHW) was notified, and a swab was taken.

That same Monday, the World Health Organization (WHO) declared the coronavirus a global pandemic.

While we waited for the swab to be processed, we all tried to busy ourselves with other work, but everyone's mind was on the test results. The lab informed the chief medical officer (CMO) first. She then told me and the permanent secretary. The patient was informed. I then notified the prime minister. This was Tuesday, March 10, 2020— the date that has come to be recognized as the beginning of the pandemic in Jamaica.

The press conference we knew was going to happen was arranged at the MOHW, New Kingston, headquarters to tell Jamaica that we had our first case. There had already been two false alarms, and the country was on edge. It was important that we communicate the news as quickly and transparently as possible.

Patient One's name was never divulged, but as soon it was announced that it was a Jamaican who arrived from the United Kingdom on March 4 for a family funeral, her family in Bull Bay knew it was her, and so did everyone else in the wider community.

Fear took hold no sooner.

That evening, a public health team was dispatched to Bull Bay, where Patient One had been staying, and contact tracing began. The public health inspectors began surveying the area using GIS (geographic information system) technology, which provided a detailed map of the family compound and the surrounding areas. The entrance to the premises on the Bull Bay main road is unremarkable, but once inside, it is a large property with around one dozen houses, extending to the sea. Some of the houses contained more than one household. Clad in personal protective equipment, the public health nurses and their teams visited each home, identified the head of household, recorded the number of people and their names, and took temperatures. Then they crossed the road to the other family home and did the same. At each household, a health alert card and a contact number were left in case persons began exhibiting symptoms, especially a fever or a cough.

The team worked late into the night, sitting with the family to compile a list of all the people who had attended the various funeral-related gatherings, including the pastor and the councillor. The taxi driver was a key contact because he had spent so much time in close proximity to her. He and his family were checked. Another team in Mocho was dispatched to cover those who Patient One had come into contact with when she visited her father.

Within the next couple of days, swabs were taken from immediate family members. Everyone in that yard and across the road was placed under mandatory home quarantine. A radius of five hundred metres was drawn around the family compound, and a larger GIS map was created, one that showed the footpaths and clusters of small houses that are invisible from the main road and which are not accounted for on existing official maps. Those maps then guided the community health aides, public health nurses, public health inspectors, and the doctors as they went door-to-door. They had to go mostly on foot, particularly to the small dwellings behind zinc fences, as the dusty paths were too small and rutted for a vehicle to traverse.

By midday on Thursday, March 12, it became clear that over thirty people had been in direct contact with Patient One. Eight people in the neighbouring household to where Patient One slept had symptoms. The taxi driver tested positive, as had people in the house where she stayed, and several people were displaying symptoms.

That evening, March 13, both Seven Miles and Eight Miles communities were placed under a two-week community quarantine—a first in Jamaica's modern history.

Patient One spent three weeks in isolation at the University Hospital of the West Indies (UHWI), in a ward that had just a couple of weeks before been converted to accommodate COVID-19 patients. She had not felt sick at all since the day she had gone to the doctor and been swabbed. Though she was asymptomatic, the discharge protocol was two negative swabs within forty-eight hours of each other.

I met Patient One the day she was discharged from hospital, on April 3. She was subdued and reticent. It seemed to me that she was still somewhat in shock that she had been the one to start off the coronavirus pandemic in Jamaica. She did not even know when or from whom she contracted the virus. The time in hospital had seemed pointless. The hospital stay was the least of it, however. Outside the hospital walls, back in the community, the real ordeal unfolded. I asked her if she had had any issues relating to stigma. She couldn't answer, so overcome with emotion.

Her family members had become the object of scorn and disdain; they, in turn, were angry with her at the disruption her illness had brought on all of them. Though the ministry never revealed any information to the public about Patient One, nor about any person who tested positive for COVID-19, Jamaica is a small place. People in the Seven Mile area, which is predominantly lower income, including a number of captured-land settlers, saw the health workers go into the home and made recordings that they posted on social media. The family was ostracized:

"People walk on the other side of the road that we live now, the shop [we had] affi lock because no one is coming. Everybody scared of us right now, but we are coping."

Other members of the family, who had no interaction with Patient One, were shunned. A child was asked to stay home by the primary school they attended:

"They said she can't come back until she brings a medical certificate, but she live miles away from us."

When the police visited the family, the officers spoke to them from across the street, out of fear:

"Four policemen came yesterday, one of the police come across and talk to us. Him ask fi wi name and where she was staying… The other three stayed across di road because dem 'seh dem doh wah dead."[1]

It was clear that what she wanted most was to get out of Jamaica and go back to England, away from the upheaval that she had unwittingly caused, back to her anonymity and her normal life.

By this time, however, Jamaica had closed its borders, as had the United Kingdom. In the three weeks since Patient One's positive test result was returned, to the day she left the hospital, the entire world had gone into lockdown. The Bull Bay community quarantine had ended, but the bitterness that had permeated her family and the community remained, and she dreaded going back there.

In the UK, the disease was raging. Prime Minister Boris Johnson, had tested positive for the virus and was in intensive care, after several weeks of dismissing the seriousness of the virus. Patient One was stuck in Jamaica, with no certainty as to when she would be able to leave. Uncertainty: one of the hallmarks of the pandemic. In those early, early days, we had no conception of what lay ahead.

---

[1] "BUZZ Exclusive: Family of Jamaica's patient zero clears the record," *Buzz*, March 11, 2020, https://buzz-caribbean.com/news/buzz-exclusive-family-of-jamaicas-patient-zero-clears-the-record/. Translation: "Four policemen came yesterday, one of the police come across and talk to us. He asked our name and where she was staying… the other three stayed across the road because, they said, they do not want to die."

On Alert |

Patient One may have been Jamaica's first diagnosed coronavirus case, and the date of that diagnosis became widely used as the beginning of the pandemic in Jamaica, but that test result did not mark the start of Jamaica's COVID-19 journey. That diagnosis marked the transition to the second stage of the epidemic. Preparations had begun some six weeks before, in January, when what came to be called COVID-19 was still thought to be just a new respiratory virus wreaking havoc in China.

December 31, 2019, was the first clear sign that we saw that there would be a problem. The Wuhan Municipal Health Commission website noted cases of "viral pneumonia" in the city, the capital of Central China's Hubei province. That same day, a media report on the ProMED website (a programme of the International Society for Infectious Diseases) carried information about the same cluster of cases of "pneumonia of unknown cause" in Wuhan.

By January 2, 2020, the World Health Organization (WHO) began to notify the Global Outbreak Alert and Response Network (GOARN) partners (major public health agencies, laboratories, sister UN agencies, international organizations, and NGOs) about the cluster of pneumonia cases in China.

On January 4, in a tweet, WHO shared the news with the world. On January 11, Chinese media reported the first death from the virus, now being called a "novel coronavirus." On January 13, the Ministry of Public Health in Thailand reported an imported case of novel coronavirus from Wuhan, the first recorded case outside of China. On January 16, the Japanese authorities delivered news of an imported case, also from Wuhan.

By this time, it was becoming clearer that the virus might be transmitted human-to-human, though the Chinese authorities reported that there was no clear evidence to support this.

It first occurred to me that the world was on the brink of something serious at the beginning of the third week of January. I had seen unofficial footage that people in Wuhan, China, where the virus first appeared, had taken with their phones. At that time, the Chinese authorities were still insisting that the virus was likely not as deadly or infectious as the SARS outbreak and was "still preventable and controllable." Yet here were videos showing catastrophic scenes of hospitals overwhelmed with sick people, videos that the Chinese government did not want the world to see.

Dr. Jacquiline Bisasor-McKenzie, Jamaica's chief medical officer, had also taken note of the virus and was watching the news out of China. For her, once the virus began to spread beyond China and appeared in Italy, which is a source country of many tourists who visit Jamaica, there was no question that this novel coronavirus was going to eventually reach Jamaica.

From the moment that we at the Ministry of Health and Wellness were in agreement that this virus was heading towards us, we were in a race against time. The immediate goal was to delay the virus's arrival in Jamaica as long as possible, in order to put the necessary measures in place. It wasn't a matter of if but when, and we needed to push that "when" back as far as we could.

The tacit consensus was that if what we saw could happen in China, a country with far more resources and a much more comprehensive public health system than Jamaica has, then a disease like that in Jamaica would be detrimental. Our under-resourced and fragmented public healthcare system was not equipped to absorb an epidemic of that scale, of a disease that appeared to be highly contagious. Furthermore, the Jamaican economy had only just stabilized after a long period of stagnation and decline and a brutal spell of economic hardship.

Infectious diseases were already a problem in Jamaica. When coronavirus came about, Jamaica was struggling with an unprecedented two-year outbreak of dengue fever in the Latin American and Caribbean Region. Over 1,000 people in 2018 contracted dengue, and 17 died.

In 2019, that number increased exponentially to 9,159, with 67 deaths. For a country as small as Jamaica, these numbers are alarmingly high. When those videos from Wuhan began to emerge in January, there were already 103 dengue cases counted and 1 death, despite months of efforts and huge expenditure of resources. We had added sixty vehicles to the eradication team's fleet and one thousand vector control workers. There was a national clean-up effort, a public education campaign, and mounted foggers. Yet dengue remained a problem.

We had to face the question: could we ever be ready for anything near the scale of what we were seeing in China? To begin with, we didn't have the numbers of healthcare workers, hospital beds, ventilators, or personal protective equipment. We had only forty functional ICU beds across a handful of public hospitals and thirty-five ventilators, which were nearly always in use.

Prioritization of cases was a regular aspect of the management of critical-care patients in Jamaica's hospitals. Even if we had more ICUs, we wouldn't have the staff to man them. We were already only at 50 to 60 percent of our specialist nursing needs in normal times. This was without factoring in the inevitable attrition from healthcare workers who would undoubtedly fall ill from the virus and those who would not come to work, whether for fear of the virus or because they had underlying conditions that made the risk too great. Our hospital waiting rooms had been one of the first-priority issues that I set out to fix when I first became minister in 2016, so I knew that they did not have the capacity to deal with a surge of sick, contagious people.

However, it was not all doom and gloom. What we did have was a robust surveillance system, as infectious diseases were not new to Jamaica. We had experience in contact tracing, most recently in 2006, when we had a malaria outbreak and some 4,000 people were infected. That system of frontline workers would prove to be invaluable in the COVID-19 response to come.

Wild Flavours |

In 2010, a Jamaican who had gone bird shooting in South America became fascinated by the monkeys he saw there. He managed to have one captured, and he smuggled it into the island to take home with him as a pet. Cute and exotic, it seemed like a good idea at the time.

But it didn't end well. The monkey attacked and bit his young son, and the child was taken to the doctor. When the man heard that the child had to be tested for rabies and Herpes B—a serious disease that can lead to encephalitis, swelling of the brain, and death—he understandably panicked. He had no idea of the danger he had put his family and the entire country in by illegally importing this wild animal into the island. Fortunately, the child was fine, and the monkey was euthanized.

The deadliest viruses of this generation have emerged from human contact with live animals. More than 80 percent of emerging human diseases in the twenty-first century originate in animals, mainly wild animals. As the world becomes increasingly urbanized and deforested, humans encroach on wildlife, and their viruses and bacteria get into human circulation.

The West African Ebola virus almost certainly was transmitted from a type of bat that resembles a flying mouse. The Asian flu pandemic that emerged from wild ducks in 1957 killed as many as two million people globally. Severe acute respiratory syndrome (SARS), which emerged in 2002–2003, may have spread from bats to humans, via masked palm civets (a wild cat) and other species in live-animal markets before it began infecting people.

The 2009 HINI influenza virus was first detected in people in the United States in April 2009. The virus was originally referred to as "swine flu" because laboratory testing showed that its gene segments

5

were similar to influenza viruses that were identified in and known to circulate among pigs.[2]

The Middle East respiratory syndrome (MERS) was a new coronavirus first reported in 2012 in Saudi Arabia, thought to have originated in Jordan. It likely came from an animal source in the Arabian Peninsula, probably a camel.[3]

The Zika virus (Zik-V), between 2016 and 2018, affected over nine thousand Jamaicans and caused over eighty deaths, including global Zik-V numbers. Though it was spread by mosquitoes, it originated in monkeys that were bitten by mosquitoes and then bit men hunting those monkeys.

Aside from people who manage to illegally get wild animals across the border, Jamaica has a strong record of keeping the island free of animal-borne diseases. We have strict border guidelines for the importation of all animals, whether dead (meat) or alive. Culturally, we do not have a tradition of eating raw meat. Indeed, we tend to overcook our meat, which would kill any pathogen (disease-causing agent) that happened to sneak in. Those border controls and cultural preferences are meaningless, however, when a human being becomes the agent of a disease, in a world where people travel extensively, all across the globe.

China is closely acquainted with deadly pathogens, mostly thought to originate in animals. A wet market is where live crocodiles, hedgehogs, deer, and other wild animals are sold. China's wet markets sell freshly slaughtered, unpackaged meat. The market conditions can set off potentially deadly contagions, as shoppers mingle in narrow spaces, with everything from live poultry to snakes.

---

[2] "H1N1 Influenza (Swine Flu) and You," Centers for Disease Control and Prevention, November 25, 2009, www.cdc.gov/h1n1flu/information_h1n1_virus_qa.htm.

[3] "Middle East Respiratory Syndrome (MERS)," Centers for Disease Control and Prevention, last updated August 2019, ww.cdc.gov/coronavirus/mers/about/index.html.

Wet markets are popular and are a central part of life in many cities. "Wild flavour" is the name given to exotic animals, which are considered more nourishing and richer in flavour than farm-grown animals. This preference for fresh meat from animals that aren't properly quarantined or come from the wild makes China susceptible to the risk of new virus outbreaks, through close animal and human contact.

•————————————•

In late December 2019, a cluster of pneumonia cases emerged in Wuhan, in Hubei province in China. The illness was unlike any that had ever been seen before and did not respond to medication. It also appeared to be highly contagious.

In early January 2020, the virus that caused this illness, first called SARS-CoV-2 (what would come to be called COVID-19), was identified.[4]

There was a wet market in Wuhan where the virus was first suspected to have emerged. The new coronavirus, it was first reported, was found in people who shopped or worked at this wet market, and the pathogen may have been transmitted to humans from live animals sold there—what is called a zoonotic source. Other scientific research later found that many of the first known patients had no direct exposure to that market.[5]

Regardless of the precise source, however, most scientists have concluded that this coronavirus originated in wildlife. How the severe acute respiratory syndrome coronavirus 2 (SARS-CoV-2), the agent responsible for the coronavirus disease 2019 (COVID-19) virus, crossed over into humans was debated throughout the pandemic.

---

[4] The name *COVID-19* was shortened from Corona Virus Disease, and the year it came about, health officials purposely avoid naming COVID-19 after a geographical location as with Ebola or Middle East, animal as with Swine flu, or group of people, so as not to stigmatize people or places.

[5] Chaolin Huang et al., "Clinical Features of Patients Infected with 2019 Novel Coronavirus in Wuhan, China," The Lancet 395, no. 10223 (2020): 497–506, https://doi.org/10.1016/S0140-6736(20)30183-5.

Beyond a consensus that it certainly originated in an animal, scientists went back and forth over which animal and how exactly the transmission occurred.

Bats and pangolins were the primary suspects. By the end of 2022, the consensus went no further than an agreement that whether or not it was a straightforward animal-to-human transmission, it was an outcome of humans' complex interaction with wildlife.

There was also a lab leak theory, which wasn't one single theory, but several explanations that had the commonality of blaming the Chinese government, through its scientific institutions, for the emergence of the virus and hence the pandemic. These explanations went from being ridiculed as conspiracy theories to being considered enough of a possibility to lead to an enquiry ordered by US President Biden.

I never assumed a lab leak of some sort, whether intentional or accidental, wasn't a possibility; there were several aspects of various theories that were plausible. The enquiry report was unable to unequivocally resolve the origin question, and many esteemed scientists agree that while the evidence points to a zoonotic source, a lab leak is not out of the realm of possibility.

The outbreak of a new disease with the potential to spread across the world had, for a long time, been inevitable, but this one happened in the worst place at the wrong time. Wuhan is a big city and a crossroads, and the time of year—the Lunar New Year and the Spring Festival holiday at the end of January—had people travelling extensively.[6] It was a peak travel season for Chinese citizens, as the full week of public holidays gives time for trips abroad.

In the first three weeks of January 2020, 81 percent of reported cases in China were from Hubei, after which most other Chinese provinces reported rapid increases in cases.

6 Jonathan Quick, "The Worst-Case Scenario for Coronavirus: Q&A with Dr. Jonathan Quick," The Guardian, March 1, 2020, www.theguardian.com/world/2020/mar/01/the-worst-case-scenario-for-coronavirus-dr-jonathan-quick-q-and-a-laura-spinney.

A travel ban in Hubei was announced on January 23, 2020, two days before the Lunar New Year holiday, but movement of individuals out of Wuhan had already started in the days before that.[7]

By January 27, about three thousand cases had been confirmed in China, and cases were also reported in Japan, South Korea, Thailand, Singapore, the United States, and Australia, all of which were thought to have been exported from China.

Jamaica announced a ban against travelers from China on January 31. This was one of the most important early decisions that we took. Shortly thereafter, having determined that a ban on other countries' travelers was necessary, we convened a meeting of several ambassadors at the Ministry of Foreign Affairs and Foreign Trade in Kingston. The purpose of the meeting was to discuss the impending travel bans and the situation in general. While I was giving the justification for bans, the building began to shake. It was a small earthquake. The meeting was cut short as we all evacuated the building. The important messages had already been conveyed, but the symbolism of that unexpected earthquake was profound: the world was facing great uncertainty and those were the first rumblings.

---

[7] Moritz U. G. Kraemer et al., "The Effect of Human Mobility and Control Measures on the COVID-19 Epidemic in China," *Science* 368 (2020): 493–497, doi:10.1126/science.abb4218.

Time and Trust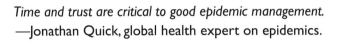

Time and trust are critical to good epidemic management.
—Jonathan Quick, global health expert on epidemics.

If an epidemic can be detected early, it makes a difference. Actions taken even a day too late can have massive repercussions. When the disease is unknown—it's new, and no one knows how it behaves— early action can appear unnecessarily cautious, and there is a risk of blowing the situation out of proportion. While erring on the side of caution may seem the most prudent choice, those errors can be very costly, particularly when the anticipated outcome doesn't manifest.

The COVID-19 pandemic and its effects worldwide were unprecedented, but the possibility of such a phenomenon was well known. Many may have thought that the idea of an unknown and highly contagious virus spreading worldwide, shutting it down, was the stuff of fiction and movies.

But public health experts globally, including in Jamaica, however, knew it was not only possible but also inevitable. For years, decades even, scientists had declared that a global pandemic was bound to happen.

In 2007, the European Molecular Biology Organization (EMBO) declared that a global pandemic like those in the movies "is a certainty, with the only uncertainties being what pathogen will cause it, when it will happen, and how well the world will cope," and that "the probability of another flu pandemic (like the Spanish flu) is 100 percent, though we cannot say when exactly."[8]

---

[8] Hunter P., "Inevitable or Avoidable? Despite the Lessons of History, the World is Not Yet Ready to Face the Next Great Plague," *EMBO Rep.* 8, no. 6 (2007): 531–534, doi:10.1038/sj.embor.7400987.

The world's growing population becoming more urban, densely populated, and exceedingly mobile across geographical boundaries all create greater opportunities for diseases to spread through air, mosquitoes, or unclean water. These can then be transported by human hosts. Because infectious agents can live in humans during their incubation period (the time between infection and the onset of symptoms), travelers can transmit an infection to another region even though they don't appear to be sick. This would turn out to be one of the most dangerous features of the COVID-19 virus. There was a long incubation period, and people with the virus were often asymptomatic but still able to infect others. Ongoing urbanization also brings humans into previously uninhabited territories, such as forests, where they are more likely to come into more frequent contact with wild animals and, inevitably, new infections.

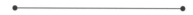

Jamaica's Ministry of Health and Wellness already had a pandemic influenza response plan, prepared in 2006 and updated in 2007, by then-chief medical officer and director, emergency, disaster management, and special services, Dr. Marion Bullock DuCasse, which was adapted to a novel coronavirus response plan. That plan was based on the principles of rapid implementation of global and national actions, guidance from the WHO, and dependence on early disease recognition, high-level political support, and transparent communication. There were also specific logistical arrangements to be put in place and protocols to be followed. Having this plan already formulated meant that we were able to proceed without delay.

The plan had four phases: 1) inter-pandemic, 2) alert phase, 3) pandemic phase, 4) and recovery phase.[9]

The inter-pandemic phase had come and gone. That was the period during which there was no active influenza virus that was posing a threat of becoming an epidemic. We were now in the alert phase,

---

[9] These are standard to most pandemic response plans.

where a new influenza had been identified in humans, and the task was to prepare for the disease coming to Jamaica.

The main elements are the following: 1) putting in place measures to detect the disease early, ensuring our laboratories had the capacity to test, 2) expanding hospital capacity especially with regard to isolation facilities and critical care, 3) and communicating with the public. We also reviewed possible containment measures for the next phases.

We were in a state of readiness from our preparedness for Ebola. An Ebola response plan was developed in 2014 during the outbreak in West Africa, at the time the largest in history. That outbreak was classified as a public health emergency of international concern and had the potential to become a global pandemic, having spread from Guinea to Liberia and Sierra Leone, with cases in Mali, Nigeria, four cases in the United States (two imported, two contacts of one of the imported cases), and single cases in four other countries.

The trust issue was less straightforward, but just as important. Jamaica is a low-trust society. Most Jamaicans do not trust each other. Almost all Jamaicans believe corruption is widespread throughout the society, and very few Jamaicans have confidence in their government and the agents of the state.[10] But virtually everything that we were going to have to do would require the cooperation of the general population to be effective, and for people to cooperate, they would have to have trust in the authorities. From the outset, this was clear. The news coming out of China about the disease was scary—so much was unknown about how it was spread, and hypotheses and rumors were rife.

The panic that rippled through the entire capital city, Kingston, when the first unsubstantiated rumour spread that there was a patient with the novel coronavirus at the University Hospital of the West Indies (before Patient One was confirmed), was evidence that the levels of awareness and fear were high.

---

[10] Lawrence Powell, "Are We Experiencing An Epidemic Of Distrust?" *Gleaner*, April 7, 2010, http://jamaica-gleaner.com/gleaner/20100407/cleisure/cleisure3.html.

On Friday, January 28, the day before the ban was announced, a patient, someone who had recently traveled to China, presented after an accident and emergency at the UHWI, in Kingston. The patient showed coronavirus symptoms, and within minutes, it seemed, all of Jamaica knew.

A test was done. It had to be sent to Trinidad and Tobago to be tested at the Caribbean Public Health Agency (CARPHA) because Jamaica did not yet have its testing capacity. The test came back negative. We had a press conference to share this with the country, the first show of our commitment to transparency to shore up trust.

Building that trust meant not only transparency but also consistency. It entailed disseminating evidence-based information in a language that could be understood by everyone and responding promptly to concerns, especially to dispel misinformation. We had to ensure that people's needs were met, whether it was patients ill with the disease, or, later, people in communities put under quarantine, or returning citizens who had to go into state quarantine. We recognized that if we were to mislead or be perceived to have misled the population, we would lose their trust and cooperation.

How that manifested was in unparalleled transparency and accountability on the part of the Jamaican state. There has never been a situation in Jamaica where the government has been so forthcoming with information, often before there is even a demand for that information. The demand was certainly there; the news media was hungry for "scoops," and the population desperate for news. This extraordinary responsiveness was manifested in the scores of advisories, the extensive use of social media platforms, dozens of press briefings, and countless radio interviews with myself and other senior ministry officials, including when the news wasn't positive, and we were likely to receive flack for mistakes or unpopular decisions. We made ourselves available to be held accountable in a way no other elected or public official has ever done.

Once the virus reached Jamaica, and we were sharing the daily updates of numbers of new cases and fatalities, I was the first to share it on my Twitter feed. A few minutes before, when I knew the update was about to be sent to me, I would post a GIF that said "loading." The responses to that initial post were themselves something to behold. People were waiting for that post even when it came late into the night. A few minutes after, I would post the update. It was a strange feeling to be the bearer of information that so many people were so invested in receiving. It was strange all around: Jamaicans were not used to such prompt transmission of information from their government, and very quickly, a new norm was established.

I eventually suspended that way of releasing the update. Some said they were glad because it was stressful; others said they missed the anxiety. Later still, the update was issued directly from the ministry's social media accounts.

Travel Ban |

On January 21, 2020, my fifty-second birthday, new coronavirus cases were reported outside of mainland China, in Taiwan, and in the US.

On January 22, the MOHW issued its first advisory. The advisory acknowledged that the MOHW was aware of the disease, that there was no case reported in Jamaica, and gave basic disease prevention hygiene tips. That same week, we began sensitizing the relevant stakeholders by sending information, alerting them to the imminent threat of the virus, and advising precautionary measures. Airport screening measures were stepped up, and enhanced surveillance implemented.

I briefed the prime minister on the situation, and by the following Monday, January 27, I made a presentation to the cabinet explaining that the disease would reach Jamaica and that resources were needed to prepare for it. Based on the MOHW technical team's advice, I suggested that we impose a travel ban against anyone coming from China. The recommendation for the ban was no small matter, and it was politically fraught, but we took the advice of the ministry's technical team nevertheless.

Jamaica's relationship with China is strong, but has to be managed with extreme care. The Jamaica-China relationship is very important to Jamaica, particularly as China was, at the time, Jamaica's largest bilateral donor and lender. All of the country's major infrastructural projects—namely, roads and hospital—were being financed by China, whether through grants or through long-term, low-interest loans.

The Chinese are extremely sensitive to anything that could be perceived as a slight on their nation's image. They are detail-oriented, and they closely scrutinize public utterances related to them.

In 2016, there was a yellow fever outbreak in parts of Africa and South America. The ministry detained several Chinese travelers who had a travel history from an area in Libya where there was a cluster among Chinese workers there, and a ban on Chinese travelers was briefly imposed. The Chinese Embassy's reaction was swift, and Jamaica took actions to appease them, including relieving ministry officials of their jobs. The cabinet's approval of such an extreme measure was an indication of the seriousness of the situation. In our fight against the new coronavirus, the decision to close the border would have political repercussions, The Chinese would not be pleased, and it could amount to a diplomatic situation. Almost immediately after the ban was announced, I was requested to attend a meeting with the ambassador. We modified the wording, but the intended policy measure—a ban on Chinese travelers—stood.

January 30, the WHO declared the outbreak a "global health emergency," an acknowledgement that the viral disease now represented a threat beyond China. We announced the ban on travelers from China on January 31. That same day, nineteen Chinese tourists landed at the Norman Manley International Airport and were refused landing privileges.

The WHO also contacted us to raise concerns about our ban. They had not yet concluded, nor had issued policy advice to members, that measures such as travel bans were necessary. The WHO found itself from the start of the pandemic in an invidious position in its attempt to balance its members' individual interests with the broader global public health interest. The organization has to be accountable and responsive to its members, who support it financially, at the same time as it should perform its role as an impartial and objective provider of evidence-informed guidance to its members.

The China travel ban brought the problem of the Jamaicans in China to the fore. There were 589 registered Jamaican nationals across China.[11]

---

[11] "No Jamaicans in China Have Contracted COVID-19." Jamaica Information Service, March 12, 2020, https://jis.gov.jm/no-jamaicans-in-china-have-contracted-covid-19/.

There had already been concerns about their welfare, particularly the 28 in Wuhan when the city was placed on lockdown on January 23.

At first, people were allowed out of their homes, but restrictions soon tightened. No travel in or out of the city was allowed, even for medical or humanitarian reasons. Inside the city, public transport was completely suspended, and cars were banned from the roads. In some areas, this was limited to outings of just one member of a family every two days in order to buy necessities. Other areas barred residents from leaving, obligating them to order food and other supplies from couriers. At the time this seemed extreme, something that could only happen in an authoritarian state. Little did we know that lockdowns would soon become the order of the day.

The expectation that the Jamaican government should "do something" was heightened by other countries evacuating their nationals from China. Foreign Affairs and Foreign Trade Minister and Senator, the Honourable Kamina Johnson Smith, issued a statement assuring Jamaicans in China that they had not been abandoned by their government in the midst of the coronavirus outbreak. At this stage, the situation was still quite surreal, and the notion that the world was on the brink of a complete cessation of movement across borders lurked, but seemed so far-fetched.

Surely, it would soon resolve. But it didn't. It continued to get more dramatic and more serious.

A Global Health Emergency |

February marked an acceleration of decisions, events, and responses. Once we entered the alert phase, we entered a time warp that we didn't emerge from for several months. Everything from that point happened quickly. Though we had the pandemic response plan, we had not had a pandemic in modern times, and so everything that had to happen was being done for the first time. Situations would arise that had to be gauged and responded to immediately, often without all the information that one would have ideally wanted.

At that point, we had no inkling of what awaited us.

Two things were immediately clear: first, regardless of resource constraints, there was no option for the public health system to not mount a robust response; and second, for the response to be effective, there would have to be effective and functional cooperation between government ministries, departments, and agencies, which did not normally happen in the course of the country's business.

The "whole-of-government" approach that had never really moved from being a pipe dream due to our lack of capacity to effect that ideal, by necessity and almost by default, became the order of the day. That cooperation was supported by a National Disaster Risk Management Committee, co-chaired by the prime minister, the Most Honourable Andrew Holness, and the minister of local government, the Honourable Desmond McKenzie, and comprised a wide cross-section of stakeholders, including members of industry, the public sector and civil society.

What we didn't know, and couldn't have known then, was that while we had gone from phase 1 to phase 3 over the course of only a few weeks, we would remain in phase 3 for the rest of 2020 and beyond. There was no pandemic plan that ever anticipated any such scenario, and Jamaica and the rest of the world were in for a shock.

Those first two weeks in February saw disturbing developments in other parts of the world, as the novel coronavirus picked up momentum. Coronavirus deaths began to be recorded outside of China, first in the Philippines, and then in California, in the United States.

Coronavirus cases started to spike in South Korea. Dr. Li Wenliang, the Chinese ophthalmologist who was one of the first to recognize the outbreak, in December 2019, died. His messages to his colleagues warning them and encouraging them to protect themselves was leaked, and because it countered the official position of the Chinese government—that the virus was not deadly and was easily controllable—he was considered a whistle-blower. He was detained by the authorities for spreading rumours, and allegedly forced to sign a statement agreeing to stop "illegal activities." Nevertheless, he continued to speak out. In the days before his death, Dr, Li did an interview with the New York Times, where he said, "If the officials had disclosed information about the epidemic earlier, I think it would have been a lot better; there should be more openness and transparency." He was only thirty-three years old.[12]

As we moved into mid-February, three Jamaicans, recently returned from China, presented with suspected coronavirus symptoms. They were put in precautionary isolation and tested, but all were negative. Meanwhile, in the rest of the world, news of the virus, which now had a name, COVID-19, from coronavirus disease 2019, continued to grow more frightening.

An outbreak was reported in Iran, where it was first denied by the government, until the deputy minister of health, one of the government's mouthpieces of the denial, tested positive for the virus. Eventually, one of the country's vice presidents, twenty-three members of Parliament,

---

[12] Andrew Green, "Li Wenliang," The Lancet, February 18, 2020, www.thelancet.com/journals/lancet/article/PIIS0140-6736(20)30382-2/fulltext.

and several other senior government officials fell ill with the virus. A senior adviser to the supreme leader died of the disease.[13]

By the end of the month, reputable experts were saying the worst-case scenario was looking increasingly likely. The disease was present on six continents, in forty-seven countries. Jamaica added South Korea, Italy, Singapore, and Iran to its list of countries with travel restrictions. The travel restrictions, as they were enacted in Jamaica, meant that all Jamaicans, permanent residents, and spouses of Jamaicans who had visited any of those countries in the previous fourteen days would be admitted, but would be subject to a health assessment and quarantine, with a possibility of being placed in state quarantine. Anyone with symptoms would be placed in isolation. As we used the terminology, quarantine was for those who had been exposed to the virus. They were to be separated from other people for a set period of time. Isolation was for anyone who had tested positive or whose symptoms were almost certainly those of the virus. All others who had travelled to those countries in the previous fourteen days would be denied entry entirely. Eight travelers were turned back. Ten other travelers, arriving from these countries, were put into a state quarantine facility, and seventy-eight were ordered to quarantine at home.

But travel into Jamaica is not only by plane. Nearly two million people land on Jamaica's shores each year on cruise ship stopovers. On February 25, 2020, the arrival of the cruise ship, the MSC *Meraviglia* at the port of Ocho Rios, was the next turning point in Jamaica's COVID-19 story.

---

[13] Kamiar Alaei and Arash Alaei, "How Iran Completely and Utterly Botched its Response to the Coronavirus," *New York Times*, March 6, 2020, www.nytimes.com/2020/03/06/opinion/coronavirus-iran.html.

Floating Petri Dish |

I knew there was a problem when I saw over a dozen missed calls and scores of WhatsApp messages on my phone. It had been charging for less than an hour, and I hadn't paid it attention. One of the missed calls was from the prime minister (PM). It was a Tuesday afternoon, and I was, as usual, in office at the ministry in New Kingston, about to head to Gordon House for the regular sitting of Parliament. I glanced at the list of missed calls—the minister of tourism, the Honourable Edmund Bartlett; the minister's senior advisor, Delano Seivwright; the head of the port authority, professor Gordon Shirley; and my permanent secretary (PS), Mr. Dunstan Bryan.

I called the PS first so I could get an understanding of what was clearly a crisis situation before I returned the PM's call.

It is standard operating procedure when any cruise vessel approaching a Jamaican port of call that the ship's command reports any illness on board to the relevant local health authorities. It also customary for health workers to board any incoming vessel to carry out an inspection. All the port health workers had been sensitized to the novel coronavirus, and so were on high alert. Not that they were unusually on high alert, I was already known to the cruise industry as a hardliner who put the country's public health before all else. Royal Caribbean's *Oasis of the Seas* had not been allowed to disembark any passengers just a year before, in January 2019, because over one hundred passengers had norovirus (the extremely contagious gastrointestinal illness). That incident led to the unusual step of the cruise line's CEO visiting Jamaica in person to express his dissatisfaction.

That morning, the MSC *Meraviglia*, an Italian cruise line whose market is primarily Europe, South America, and southern Africa, arrived in Ocho Rios, St. Ann, from Miami. The ship was carrying 4,500 passengers and 1,600 crew members. When the health authorities boarded the vessel, they discovered a crew member had been placed in isolation on board. That crew member had a travel history to a country with the novel coronavirus and showed symptoms associated with the disease: cough, fever, and associated muscle pains. The ship's captain had not reported this before arriving, and the ship was ordered to remain at sea. All of this was creating a stir, prompting urgent communications between the cruise line's principals and government officials, hence all the attempts to reach me to get a better understanding of exactly what was happening and what could possibly be done.

I called the prime minister and shared with him all that I had been briefed on, after which I called the minister of tourism.

This was such a big deal because the cruise industry is considered to be a mainstay of Jamaica's tourism sector, which itself is a key income generator and provider of jobs. In 2019, 1.8 million cruise visitors came to Jamaica, generating approximately US$3.3 billion, a growth of some 300 percent over a ten-year period.[14] The growth in the Caribbean cruise sector resulted in the region having more than 35 percent of all cruise vacations globally.[15] The government's intention was to grow cruise shipping, and several multimillion-dollar investments had been made in upgrading and expanding port facilities across the island. On the face of it, a minister of health had no business interfering in the smooth running of this crucial sector.

Four days later, on Friday, February 29, the *Costa Luminosa*, another Italian cruise ship (whose corporate parent is Carnival Cruises), docked in Ocho Rios. After several hours, the health officers determined that though there were four people on board with flu-like symptoms, they hadn't been in a country of COVID-19-interest. But the Italian passengers were barred from coming off the ship. By then, the coronavirus was ravaging northern Italy, and Italian travelers had already exported the virus to about fifteen countries. The public

---

[14] "Jamaica's Cruise Tourism Earns $22.6 Billion," Jamaica *Observer*, March 7, 2019, https://www.jamaicaobserver.com/2019/03/07/jamaicas-cruise-tourism-earns-22-6-billion/.

[15] David Jessop, "Reassessing the Role of Cruise Tourism," Jamaica *Gleaner*, September 15, 2019, http://jamaica-gleaner.com/article/business/20190915/david-jessop-reassessing-role-cruise-tourism.

reaction ranged from outrage and condemnation to full support. Were we destroying our cruise industry because of a virus which might not be all that serious? Or were we right to assert our sovereignty and protect the health of Jamaicans?

A few days later, a virtual meeting was convened by then-CARICOM chair, Barbados prime minister, Mia Mottley. Attending were Caribbean Community (CARICOM) health ministers, heads of cruise lines, Pan American Health Organization (PAHO), and CARPHA.

CARICOM is the regional integration organization of the English-speaking Caribbean, Haiti, and Suriname. Founded in 1973 as a customs union, the organization has struggled to fulfill its objective of bringing its members together as a single market and economy, and sometimes has strayed from its stated goal of a unified foreign policy. PM Holness joined that meeting, as did St. Lucia's prime minister, Allan Chastanet. Those of us in Jamaica all convened in a conference room at Jamaica House, the Office of the Prime Minister. I was taken aback by the presence of the cruise interests in what I thought should have been a governmental-level discussion, but PM Mottley had already invited them, and there they were.

The meeting sought to arrive at a common position on cruise ships in the context of the virus. From the cruise lines' perspective, Jamaica was the bad guy in the virtual room, having been the first to refuse a ship. PM Mottley appeared to be trying to accommodate the cruise lines, understandably given cruise shipping's importance to Barbados's tourism and economy. Eight hundred thousand cruise visitors annually go into the port of Barbados, a country of just under three hundred thousand people, but the cruise shipping aspect of Barbados's tourism industry, which in 2019 contributed 36 percent of the country's GDP, had been in decline for years.[16]

---

[16] "Barbados Contribution of Travel and Tourism to GDP - Percent of GDP," Knoema World Atlas, undated, https://knoema.com/atlas/Barbados/topics/Tourism/Travel-and-Tourism-Total-Contribution-to-GDP/Contribution-of-travel-and-tourism-to-GDP-percent-of-GDP.

One of PM Mottley's first actions as head of government was to create a national cruise development commission, with a mission to "establish Barbados as the premier cruise destination in the Caribbean and Latin American cruise region."[17] When, just months after following the commission's recommendations to pursue new cruise marketing and product development initiatives, this shock happened, it was not surprising she would be anxious to protect the investment that had already been made and the prospects those investments were intended to yield.

The representative from MSC *Meraviglia* began by laying into Jamaica about how much money they lost when they were refused permission to land, after which Cayman also refused them: US$5 million, he said. That set the meeting off on a negative footing, which PM Mottley valiantly tried to reign in and steer in a more positive direction. Carnival threatened to pull out of Jamaica completely, which was significant, since they represented about 80 percent of Jamaica's cruise ship arrivals. While we were all on the call, other health ministers were privately messaging me to say they supported me, but no one spoke up, except PM Chastanet. His stated position was to try to find a balance between protecting people and accommodating the industry.

We eventually agreed on a protocol to be established around cruises, but individual countries reserved the right to make adjustments. This was a typical CARICOM outcome: spend hours talking about something, and then come to an agreement to which no one is bound.

I went into the meeting a bit cynical because I am not much of a fan of cruise ship tourism for Jamaica. I have never been convinced that the industry contributes much to Caribbean development, government revenues, or the local economy. I have long been wary of the detrimental environmental impacts on our vulnerable marine ecosystems, particularly in the context of climate change. I disliked the

---

[17] National Cruise Development Commission (Barbados), "A New Dawn for Cruise Tourism in Barbados: Final Report," February 2019, www.barbadosparliament.com/uploads/sittings/attachments/1b7db6242eb53d0e5f859e872bf7e74a.pdf.

way the cruise lines wielded influence and power over local officials and businesses.

That aside, the cruise ships were floating petri dishes for COVID-19, as they have been for any contagious respiratory or gastrointestinal infection or virus. Thousands of passengers and crew members from different parts of the world, with varying levels of immunity, in a confined space, mixing intimately and intensely for a prolonged period of time—ideal contagious virus transmission conditions. Coronavirus, which was spread through droplets of mucus or saliva that had landed on surfaces, or that had travelled from one person to another, could be infectious without direct contact with a carrier.

Regardless of my own biases, as the person in charge of protecting Jamaicans' health, I was not satisfied that the cruise lines had adequately addressed infection prevention and control measures, and I felt they were a danger to the country as a means by which the virus would enter the island.

Nevertheless, I found myself on a plane on Thursday, March 4, with the minister of tourism and the CMO, going to Miami to meet with the cruise lines in person. I was uncomfortable going to them to meet on their turf rather than them come to us. However, given how high the stakes were, I welcomed the opportunity to clarify Jamaica's position. I asked that the attorney general, Marlene Malahoo-Forte to accompany us because we needed a lawyer. A Port Authority of Jamaica official also went.

Our first meeting was with Carnival. It did not go well. They wanted a guarantee that their ships would be allowed to dock and not be turned away at the last minute. I let the CMO do most of the talking. She could not agree to that and insisted it be on a ship-by-ship basis. They refused to agree to provide temperature logs, which for us was a red-line issue. I felt like we were under interrogation, and the sense of entitlement from the other side of the table was disheartening. Despite the minister of tourism trying his best to reach a compromise, the meeting ended with no agreement. As we were leaving, St. Lucia's prime minister, Chastanet, was entering the building.

Next meeting was with MSC *Meraviglia*. This also did not get off to a good start. Leading the meeting was the same executive chairman who had been so obnoxious to me in the CARICOM Zoom meeting. He started off by apologizing for his behaviour in that meeting, but it was obvious that it was insincere, and I told him so. He didn't take kindly to that. The discussion began, and he suddenly stopped talking. We were all confused. He gestured towards the CMO who was looking at her phone and condescendingly said, "I will wait until you are finished with what you're busy with, dear." I took offence to that, and told him so.

The tensions at that point were high, and his CEO called a five-minute break so they could have a private discussion. When they left the room, our team had the opportunity to discuss our own differences among ourselves and how we should proceed. My position was that the cruise executive was being disrespectful, and I would not accept that. When the MSC chairman came back in the room, he had a bottle of tablets with him. He put it on the table and told us that it was his blood pressure medicine, and he had just spoken to his wife and told her that he had finally met someone else who could make him need to take his tablets as she did. The attempt at levity worked. After that, we were able to come to an agreement.

After the meeting, back in my hotel room, I turned on the television. The drama of the *Grand Princess* cruise ship was unfolding before the world. The ship was docked off the coast of Oakland, California, as it had been refused landing, even though it had US citizens onboard. There were twenty-one people onboard confirmed to have COVID-19. They had not been informed of their positive test results and heard it along with the rest of the world when US Vice President Michael Pence announced it on national television.

On live television, I watched a helicopter dropping test kits and supplies to the ship. The *Grand Princess* was the first cruise ship spectacle, with

3,500 passengers and crew forced to idle for days off the Northern California coast. The passengers were forced to stay in their rooms for three weeks after the two-week cruise was to have ended. For the US public, the *Grand Princess* became a symbol of America's fear of coronavirus, but at that moment, for me, it confirmed that we were correct in our position.

These were not isolated incidents. The *Diamond Princess* also came to the world's attention as, at one point, the ship had the most COVID-19 cases—over 700—in any one place outside of China. It went into lockdown, with some 3,700 people onboard, and was quarantined in Yokohama, Japan, for two weeks. An eighty-year-old Hong Kong man who had been on the ship had fallen ill with the virus. Though he was taken off the ship early and the cruise continued, the virus lingered behind and spread. When the cruise was supposed to have ended, the passengers were instead confined to their cabins for two weeks' quarantine. Eventually, there were 634 infections and two deaths on the ship. Untested passengers and passengers who got negative results but later were found to have the virus left the ship and walked free into Tokyo, onto public transportation, or to wherever else they were heading.[18]

Closer to home, Trinidad and Tobago had its own experience with the cruise ship as a super incubator. The *Costa Favolosa*, a sister ship to the *Costa Luminosa*, the second ship that we had not allowed to dock, set sail on March 7. The ship, which can accommodate 2,968 passengers, did a weekly Caribbean cruise, departing from and returning to Martinique; that fateful sailing had seventy-two Trinidadians onboard. Early in the cruise, two passengers were confirmed to have COVID-19. A few days later, there were nine confirmed cases. The ship made its way back to Guadeloupe on March 14, but then became stranded, as it was not given permission to land because of the presence of the virus on board. Eventually, the Trinidad and Tobago government chartered a flight, and sixty-eight nationals were returned to the island,

---

[18] "On Japan's Virus-Hit Cruise Ship, Room Service Comes with a Knock and a Temperature Check," *The New York Times*, February 22, 2020, www.nytimes.com/2020/02/22/world/asia/coronavirus-japan-cruise-ship.html.

where they were immediately put in quarantine. Forty-seven of the group tested positive for COVID-19, taking Trinidad's numbers from seventeen to sixty-five in one fell swoop. Trinidad's second recorded COVID-19 death was of a man who had been on that cruise. Ten of the Dominican Republic's first few dozen COVID-19 cases were later reported to have been linked to the ship's stop there on March 10.

Any notion that we were overreacting was quickly dismissed, as cruise ships began to be denied entry at ports around the world. Despite reassurances that cruising was safe and would continue regardless, cruise shipping was on its back foot. Some public health experts went so far as to say that cruise ships had played a significant role in spreading the virus around the world.[19]

The day after those two difficult meetings in Miami, a Carnival executive reached out to me. She apologized for how the meeting had transpired. "We want to find a way to meet your demands," she said. It ended up that we came to the same agreement with Carnival as we had with MSC.

The Costa Luminosa, the second cruise ship that posed an issue when we wouldn't let the Italians disembark, had gone from Jamaica to Cayman, where an ill passenger was medically evacuated. That person later tested positive for COVID-19 and died. As the ship continued to sail, an Italian passenger was the first to fall ill on board. Fourteen more Costa Luminosa passengers later died from COVID-19. Had we allowed that ship to disembark all its passengers, Jamaica would likely have had the coronavirus come into the island far sooner than it eventually did.

For all the fuss that was made about the cruise ships, and all the time and energy that sorting that out consumed, it soon became clear that it was wasted effort. One short week later, all those discussions and meetings were moot. On Friday, March 13, all major cruise lines

---

[19] "Coronavirus on a Cruise Ship: Disease Traced Back to One Passenger," The Washington Post, April 25, 2020, www.washingtonpost.com/graphics/2020/politics/cruise-ships-coronavirus/.

announced they would cease US sailings for at least the next thirty days, in an effort to stop the spread of coronavirus. It would in fact be fifteen months before the no-sail order issued by the US Centers for Disease Control and Prevention was lifted, and any cruise ships ventured out again.

Once the cruise ships all halted operations, they were no longer a problem for us. Or so we thought. The cruise ships would soon return as one of our biggest challenges.

The Spread Begins |

The cruise ship drama behind us, preparations continued on the ground in Jamaica. Going into March, attention was directed to the build out of isolation wards at hospitals around the island, sourcing PPE, acquiring ventilators, and training staff. Our projections, based on epidemiological models and the available information, was that up to 1.6 million Jamaicans, more than half the population, could be impacted by the disease, but fewer than 400 would likely develop serious problems. That number was mind-boggling, and terrifying. How would we ever combat something with that potential?

Our eyes, as were the world's, were on Italy, which had taken over the spotlight from China as the global epicentre of this novel coronavirus. They were one of the first countries outside of China to have confirmed cases, when two people tested positive in Rome on January 31. (Research later showed the virus was most likely present in the US as early as December.)[20] A sudden spike a few weeks later, from 5 cases to a 150, in the north of the country was the beginning of a sustained surge that, in the first phase of the pandemic, would make Italy one of the worst-hit countries in the world.

At the time, we didn't realize there would be more than one phase. We thought that what we were witnessing in March was THE pandemic.

In Bergamo, a northern province with just under 1 million people, there are usually fewer than 1,000 deaths each month. In March 2020, nearly 6,000 people died. The scale of death was akin to that seen in extreme famine or war.[21]

---

[20] "Antibodies to Severe Acute Respiratory Syndrome Coronavirus 2 (SARS-CoV-2) in All of US Research Program Participants, 2 January to 18 March 2020," *Clinical Infectious Diseases*, 74 (4), 15 February 2022, 584–590, https://academic.oup.com/cid/article/74/4/584/6294073.
[21] Allison McCann, Jin Wu and Josh Katz, "How the Coronavirus Compares With 100 Years of Deadly Events," *New York Times*, June 10, 2020, www.nytimes.com/interactive/2020/06/10/world/coronavirus-history.html.

By March 9, the entire country was placed under one of the strictest lockdowns anywhere in the world, in that first phase of the pandemic. It would come to include the closure of all factories and halting of all non-essential production. At one point, Italy was counting 6,500 new cases a day, and the country's healthcare system was strained. Only patients with the most severe cases were admitted to the hospital, and horror stories emerged about doctors being forced to choose who would live and who would die because they simply could not attend to everyone. The images, footage, and stories were beyond imagination.

The lessons from Italy were clear, and we paid attention.

At the outset, the spread of the virus in Italy did not appear to be a crisis, and it was not treated as one by either policy-makers or the public. Despite scientists' warning of a potential catastrophe, people were skeptical, and politicians were deliberately shaking hands in public to make a point that people should not panic.

What Italy showed the world was that not only does the virus multiply and spread exponentially and rapidly, but that not acting quickly also increases the exponent and fuels its acceleration. From Italy, we could see that the most effective time to take action was extremely early, when the threat appeared small, before there were any cases. The risk was that if the intervention worked, it would appear in retrospect as if the strong actions were an overreaction. But the risk of not acting, as we saw, was deleterious.[22]

Spain too was in the spotlight, as they became the country with the fastest rate of coronavirus contagion in the world.[23] They imposed a nationwide lockdown on March 14. The health system was so overwhelmed that Madrid, the worst-hit city, had to commission

---

[22] Gary P. Pisano, Raffaella Sadun, and Michele Zanini, "Lessons from Italy's Response to Coronavirus," *Harvard Business Review*, March 27, 2020, https://hbr.org/2020/03/lessons-from-italys-response-to-coronavirus.

[23] Raphael Minder, "Spain Becomes Latest Epicenter of Coronavirus After a Faltering Response," *New York Times*, March 13, 2020, www.nytimes.com/2020/03/13/world/europe/spain-coronavirus-emergency.html.

an ice skating rink as a temporary morgue, as the spread of the disease and the pace of deaths exceeded capacity. Spain, with France and Germany, were added to Jamaica's travel restrictions list. Spain and Italy's experiences were stark examples of the necessity for governments to take strict measures early to combat the virus's spread. We were paying attention.

And finally, our first case was confirmed on Tuesday, March 10. The next day, March 11, our second case of COVID-19 was confirmed. Like the first case, the woman had also travelled from the United Kingdom. Both women were in isolation at the University Hospital of the West Indies, and contact tracing began immediately.

Patient One had been the index case for eight other cases. Patient Two worked at the United States Embassy in Kingston, and several of the employees self-quarantined.

A day later, the embassy closed completely and announced that it had flown in a team from the US to sanitise its premises. The Bank of Nova Scotia New Kingston branch was also closed and sanitised as Patient Two had been there the Monday morning before going to work at the embassy. J Wray & Nephew, a rum distiller, suspended operations at its Spanish Town Road location because one of its contractors had been in close contact with her. None of the workplaces ended up having any workers test positive for COVID-19. Indeed, Patient Two did not transmit the virus to any other person that we became aware of. We did not know it then, but these were the first iterations of how the pandemic would disrupt businesses and day-to-day life. One single positive case and an organisation with hundreds of staff, serving thousands of people a needed service, brought to a halt.

While having confirmed that the virus was in Jamaica meant we were finally out of the limbo of the waiting game, it also meant that we had truly entered a new phase of the pandemic and the response, and the rest of March brought rapid changes to the lives of all Jamaicans.

My daily routine and work were by now upended, as was that of the Ministry of Health and Wellness, as was for the entire country. The ministry's work programme was essentially suspended, as all resources were now being dedicated to the pandemic response. Regular MOHW staffers were put on a 24/7 roster. An emergency operations committee (EOC), a standard measure in any national emergency, such as a hurricane, was convened. It met twice a day, at 7:30 am and 3:00 pm in a combined in-person and Zoom meeting. (After the outbreak, at the MOHW, almost all participants attended remotely due to safety concerns.)

The EOC was the main forum in which information was shared across all sections of the MOHW, and the regional health authorities. (Jamaica's public health system is decentralized and administered by four regional health authorities, each with oversight and management of three to four of the country's fourteen parishes.) It was the control centre for coordinated response to the emergency, where all relevant information was tallied, logged, disseminated, and discussed.

Epidemiology gave numbers of cases and observed trends. The clinical status of the cases was given. The situation at the quarantine sites, including security issues, was reported on; the lab gave details on tests and testing. There were updates on pharmaceutical supplies, and the meetings sometimes went on for several hours.

Aside from the MOHW's EOC, there was also a National EOC, headed by the Office of Disaster Preparedness and Emergency Management (ODPEM), which served a similar function but across all the national entities, such as the Jamaica Constabulary Force (JCF, the police), the Jamaica Defense Force (JDF, the army), and all the other state agencies that were part of the response.

On the evening of March 10, the day the first case was announced, I assembled a COVID-19 advisory team to assist the ministry in its planning and coordination as it tackled the disease. It was comprised of top business leaders, civil society leaders, a former commissioner of police, as well as a few scientists. They acted as a sounding board for how the public health and technical aspects of managing the virus translated to the reality of Jamaica and gave feedback that was then transmitted to the team at the MOHW. It was also an information source for me as I then had a fuller picture to undergird the briefings, I gave the prime minister and the cabinet.

A cabinet subcommittee was formed and chaired by the prime minister. Ministers whose portfolios were directly involved in the pandemic response—local government, foreign affairs, finance, national security, education, tourism, and transport—were made members. That was where the detailed discussion towards decision-making took place, and those meetings lasted hours.

By March 12, we had had eight confirmed-positive cases. Five had travelled to Jamaica via the United Kingdom, while two were close contacts of Patient One. On that same day, the prime minister announced the closure of all schools for two weeks, starting Friday, March 13. He also announced a two-week ban on some public gatherings, and that a permit would be required for all others. On March 13, Jamaica was declared a disaster area, which meant that the legal framework now existed for certain extraordinary actions to be taken, including the sequestering of state resources to respond to the pandemic. Travel restrictions were placed on the United Kingdom, effective March 14. From that point, the government restricted people's movements more and more, bit by bit.

On March 16, it was mandated that non-essential workers in both the public and private sectors work from home for the next seven days. A new restriction for public gatherings of no more than twenty persons was put in place. Social distancing, later called physical distancing, was introduced as a rule, where people were to maintain a distance of three to four feet from each other. (It later went to six feet.) Bars and nightclubs were ordered closed for one week, with the police empowered to enforce the measures.

Events began to be cancelled in Jamaica and around the world. The first was the annual ISSA/GraceKennedy Boys and Girls Athletics Championship (Champs), which was to take place from March 24 to 28. This was just the second time in 110 years that there wouldn't be any Champs since its inaugural staging in 1910. The first time Champs was cancelled was in 1944, due to World War II. The Penn Relays, which had been contested uninterrupted since 1895 and celebrated its 125th consecutive running in 2019, was also canceled. For many Jamaicans, it was the cancelation of these events that brought home how serious the situation was.

When, on March 20, Jamaica closed its air and sea ports to incoming passenger traffic for two weeks (to become effective the following day, March 21), the panic was so great that it had to be delayed by three days until Tuesday, March 24. The delay was largely to allow Jamaicans who worked overseas, like seamen, to return home. A couple days later, all persons sixty-five or old and older were ordered to remain home, all public sector employees sixty-five years old and older were made to work from home, and the limit for public gatherings was reduced to ten persons.

By the end of March, Jamaica was a different place. The entire country grew quiet. No one was going anywhere. There were hardly any cars on the road. It was how the place gets when a hurricane is imminent—everyone waiting for it to come—except that no hurricane was on the horizon. The quiet persisted for days, then for weeks. People were encouraged to "*tan a yuh yaad*" (stay indoors), but unlike many other countries around the world, including in the Caribbean, there was never a complete national lockdown in that initial phase. That would come much later.

Looking back, it seems almost comical that those things were announced with time spans that suggested they might be lifted in a week or two weeks, when most of them were still in effect a year and more later. To think that when schools were ordered closed, it was for a period of two weeks. It was nearly two years before they reopened, in January 2022, and even then only partially.

In those first few months, the public health imperatives of the COVID-19 response were the government's priority. Restricting people's movements was one important measure, what would come to be called NPI (non-pharmaceutical intervention). The other intervention was to treat the people who did get sick, despite the NPIs.

Virtually every containment measure that the MOHW recommended was adopted by the cabinet. No expense was spared. The health and stability of the economy, relative to previous years in Jamaica, allowed for these massive, unplanned expenditures. About 6 billion Jamaican dollars (US$39 million) was allocated for the Ministry of Health and Wellness for its response efforts, some 10 percent more than it would have obtained without COVID-19. Within this, there was J$775 million (US$5 million) in financial support to the health authorities; infrastructure upgrades of more than J$89 million (nearly US$600,000), including equipping hospitals with an additional sixty-three intensive-care and high-dependency units; J$1.7 billion on medical equipment, such as personal protective gear and COVID-19 test kits; and more than J$500 million to procure prescription drugs. Several facilities across the island were retrofitted to quarantine and/or isolate and care for persons who were suspected or confirmed to have COVID-19.

What money could not buy, in that short term, was greater capacity in the public health system, in terms of sustainably staffing all these rollouts and bridging some of the pre-existing gaps. These capacity issues would show up over and over as weaknesses in the pandemic response.

Money could neither buy information nor guarantee that the information we did have was correct. A predominant feature of the pandemic was the constant chase for information and the processing of that information. In the first year, it was information about the virus, as each day brought better understanding of its nature and effects. It soon emerged that the new virus was not as pathogenic—causing severe illness—as the similar pneumonia-related diseases MERS and SARS. The initial estimates were that the total number of deaths from the yet-to-be-identified disease accounted for less than 3 percent of those afflicted.

Most of those who died had underlying health conditions, such as hypertension, diabetes, or cardiovascular disease that compromised their immune systems. In a country where non-communicable diseases (NCDs) are the leading cause of death and where NCDs are becoming more prevalent, this aspect of the disease's etiology was a cause of concern for Jamaica. In Jamaica, NCDs account for the top 5 leading causes of death. One in three Jamaicans has hypertension, and one in eight has diabetes. The disease burden of NCDs in Jamaica is heavy.

Even the knowledge about the extent of the virus's contagion—it was highly contagious—evolved over time. It was thought to pass directly from person to person by respiratory droplets: the tiny drops of mucous and saliva that leave the mouth when talking, coughing, or sneezing. Then it was thought to be transmitted through contact and via objects and materials. such as clothes, furniture and utensils. Further along in the pandemic, the research suggested that contaminated surfaces posed far less risk than aerosolized transmission.

What was unequivocal was that the greatest danger at that point was its rapid spread and the healthcare system being overwhelmed. Large numbers of people ill at once, even if only a few were severely ill, would overwhelm any healthcare system. This happened in many places around the world, even in the world's richest countries. These were the challenges of the novel coronavirus that we knew of in those early stages.

Nurse Shettlewood |

Whenever I go on holiday, there's an outbreak of a disease, and I have to come back to work. Nurse Charmaine Vassell-Shettlewood, senior public health nurse and in-service coordinator at the Kingston and St. Andrew (KSA) Health Department, was a national treasure. If I were to single out any one person or group to whom Jamaica owes its success with controlling the spread of the coronavirus in the first critical phase, it would be her and her team of public health workers— the community health aides, public health inspectors, the public health nurses, and the health education officers. They were quite literally the foot soldiers who did the ground work of the contact tracing and surveillance, which were the critical aspects in the management of the disease's spread in the beginning.

Nurse Vassell-Shettlewood had taken forty days of long-overdue leave on February 24, 2020, but just as the rest of the world was watching the new coronavirus, so was she, and so she was expecting the call in early March asking her to come back and do the essential, important work of contact tracing.

Contact tracing is a public health tool employed in the management and control of infectious disease outbreaks. Timely deployment of contact tracing, together with other non-pharmaceutical interventions, can mitigate and suppress infectious disease spread by tracking and attempting to break chains of transmission. Contact tracing has been used, around the world, to handle tuberculosis, measles, HIV, Ebola, and malaria, among other infectious illnesses. Nurse Shettlewood was needed to manage the troops to do the necessary work of surveying an area, going door-to-door, interviewing members of households, doing health checks, giving people information, recording everything, and then going back to follow up.

Nurse Shettlewood had been a nurse in the public health system for over twenty years, and she led the contact tracing and quarantine measures in the malaria outbreak of 2006, the Ebola threat in 2014, and several measles scares. She had been a member of the team that prepared for the possible introduction and spread of H1N1 and SARS. And many of those times, she had been on holiday and had to cut her vacation short to lead the efforts.

In her regular duties, she was in charge of eight health centres in the Kingston and St. Andrew area, but in the 2020 COVID-19 pandemic response, she was the first person on the ground in Bull Bay, where Patient One had been staying and where a number of people had contracted the virus from said patient, ultimately leading to the first community quarantine in Jamaica. She managed and coordinated the hundreds of healthcare workers who did the ground work in the communities under surveillance. She also trained the healthcare workers for the specific tasks they were to do, as well as the ongoing on boarding of the new recruits. From March, amid the thousands of people hired to work on the COVID-19 pandemic, some five hundred people were trained as contact tracers.

Nurse Shettlewood was one of a cadre of senior public health nurses who were on the frontlines across Jamaica during the COVID-19 pandemic response. And while she and others had experience with other infectious diseases, COVID-19 dwarfed them all. It demanded longer hours and fewer days off, and because this virus was so contagious, most public health workers had to isolate themselves from their families when they were off work to reduce the risk of spreading it should they contract it:

"We came into nursing because we wanted to help. Never did we think we would live to see a disease that is impacting the entire world. This is something we must do, and we do it for our country."

Contact tracing is like detective work. The first interview is with the index case. Where did you go? Who did you see? When? What kind of interaction did you have with that person? Then they have to go and find all of those people, while bearing in mind that the person might not be telling the truth. There are techniques to catch people who may have "misremembered" their movements. Then there is an interview with the secondary person, the closest contact to the index case, and the same routine is followed.

The contact tracers work with a map that has been prepared by the public health inspectors assigned to the task. This was what Cameron Bennett had signed up for. He spent twenty years as a public health officer, the last few in Trelawny, a rural parish where public health officers' work was largely comprised of visiting food retailers to ensure they had their food handlers' permits up to date. Now, he was traversing the hidden footpaths of a community where two dozen households could be hidden behind a clump of bushes, creating the map for the subsequent surveillance by the other members of the public health team.

Cameron used a variety of mapping apps for the first time in his work. He had taught himself GIS mapping and enjoyed it as a hobby for several years. Between his smartphone and the tablet that had been customized to do the map, he established a radius of 250 metres from ground zero, the larger of the two households where Patient One had stayed for the five days between arriving from England and going into isolation. It soon became clear that there were a number of households and business places that were just outside the 250-metre radius, and some that were close enough to the radius that it would have been impractical to exclude them. Might as well broaden the radius to 500 metres, he thought. His higher-ups agreed.

These were the people on Jamaica's COVID-19 frontline. They were the foot soldiers—the ones who worked the longest hours, did some of the most important work, and put themselves at great risk. Nurse Shettlewood and Mr. Bennett exemplified the commitment, skill, and professionalism that despite Jamaica's under-resourced public health system, carried Jamaica through the first phase of the COVID-19 pandemic to far better outcomes than anyone could have reasonably expected.

Charmaine Vassell-Shettlewood passed away in September 2022. I felt her loss personally, given how critical she was at that early stage of the pandemic. Amidst a lifetime of good works, she will always be remembered, never forgotten, as one of the brave leaders of Jamaica's pandemic response.

COVID Conversations |

We started out with daily press briefings, then moved to briefings a few times a week. By the end of March, we had settled into biweekly press briefings. These would come from Jamaica House, the Office of the Prime Minister, and from the ministry's emergency operations centre. The prime minister would make the big announcements, such as extending the border closure, announcing a community quarantine, or declaring a curfew. I would present the latest numbers and give relevant information about the numbers. The CMO, Dr. Bisasor-McKenzie, and sometimes the permanent secretary, Dunstan Bryan, would bring more information, usually more technical, about the state of the disease in the country and the measures being taken to contain it. Various ministers would make presentations, usually regarding the measures their portfolio ministries were taking or were going to take. These press conferences would last as long as two hours to answer all the media's questions.

These events were part of the effort to meet the need to communicate, placate, respond to publicly-issued challenges, and maintain confidence in the government. The approach wasn't welcomed by everyone; one of Jamaica's most well-respected journalists tweeted midway through a press briefing in early April:

"These statements at these #COVID19 pressers can be easily condensed and made in a very few minutes. There is very little new at each briefing. No need for these long, drawn-out statements."

But surveys later showed that Jamaicans got most of their information about the pandemic from the televised press briefings. They were also watched with keen interest throughout the Caribbean region, including by government officials, and by Jamaicans in the diaspora, who were monitoring the situation in Jamaica very closely.

The level of transparency and the responsiveness of the government was noteworthy. Jamaica enjoys one of the highest levels of press freedom in the world, but this was an entirely new standard of openness. The prime minister's social media channels and my own were used to transmit information throughout the day, often within minutes of any new development. Outside of the media briefings, I tried to reach audiences that generally don't listen to mainstream news and did an Instagram live with Spice, the popular Jamaican dancehall singer and personality, and Kevin Downswell, an evangelist and gospel singer with tens of thousands of followers on social media. This was Crisis Communications 101: reach the people where they are. People wanted information, and it was important to keep fear at bay. At the same time, we wanted to prepare people for what was expected, which was a high infection rate, hospitalizations, and deaths, so they would be forewarned.

Fake news was a problem. There was a rise in false information or hoaxes related to COVID-19 being spread globally through various media, including social media. Rumours and gossip were shared incautiously, especially on WhatsApp, Jamaica's favoured messaging platform. These often included misinformation about the origin and spread of the virus, false cures or treatments, and conspiracy theories. Everyone was an expert. We had to be the authoritative voice and not leave space for speculation to spread. So much work went into fighting misinformation, throughout the pandemic.

Coming Home to Die |

Mr. S knew he was dying. He was coughing and feeling weak. The seventy-nine-year-old, who suffered from several non-communicable diseases, made it clear to his family that he didn't feel he had much time left. He wished to return to Jamaica as soon as possible to make adjustments to his will, and he did not wish to die in the United States. He had lived in the US for decades, worked and made a living, and raised a family there, but Jamaica was his home.

The unprecedented closure of national borders and cessation of international travel did much more than stop the movement of the virus and allow countries to attempt to contain it within their geographical borders. For people who were living in a place where they weren't born, it forced a reckoning of the meaning of home. Particularly for those who had left Jamaica in search of better opportunities, Jamaica wasn't looking so bad after all. Our low numbers of cases and deaths would also have been attractive.

Mr. S travelled from New York with his wife, son, and grandson. They arrived in Jamaica on Thursday March 12, 2020, at around midnight, on a JetBlue flight. Relatives picked them up from Norman Manley International Airport, and with no cars on the road, they soon arrived at their home in Corn Piece, Hayes, in Clarendon, at 2:30 am.

That weekend, Mr. S had several visitors from other homes within the community, including family members from two other households nearby. All was well until a dispute on Sunday, after which his health declined rapidly.

On Monday, March 16, he was taken to Lionel Town Hospital. By this time, he had a fever, cough, shortness of breath, and joint pain; it was clear he was a suspected COVID-19 case and was taken from there to the Mandeville Regional Hospital, where he was placed in isolation. A first test was done, which was negative, but his presentation was so severe that a second test was done. The result of that test—positive for COVID-19—was confirmed just after noon on Wednesday, March 18. But he seemed to be improving. At 3:00 pm, he was prepared for transfer to the University Hospital of the West Indies for intensive care. He had just been loaded into the ambulance when he died.

Mr. S's determination to come home to die, perfectly understandable in normal times, had immense repercussions during the time of COVID-19. All told, Mr. S's infection was transmitted to seven other people, including his son who made the *Observer* newspaper front page when he threatened to take legal action against the government for lying that his father had COVID-19 when he only had pneumonia. (He did die of pneumonia, brought on by the COVID-19 virus.) The community of Corn Piece was put under a two-week quarantine. One of his family members who broke the quarantine and frequented the nearby community of Portland Cottage transmitted the infection to someone there and nearly led to another quarantine.

The meaning of home—this was something the COVID-19 pandemic brought a new understanding about. Never before had the inability to get home made it so clear how important it was to be able to be there. And to insist on going home to take your last breath, in the midst of a global pandemic, showed just how significant the place one calls home is to a person's soul. Mr. S got his dying wish, but in doing so, there were so many consequences for his family and for the country.

Mr. S and the people who caught the virus were among the steadily climbing number of "positives," as we had come to call them, that we saw that March. The first healthcare worker contracted the virus, though not on the job; she was a contact of a confirmed case. For almost every positive, we knew where they had contracted the virus. Except for the mystery cases. In the reporting, these were called "local transmission, not epidemiologically linked." By the end of June, there were thirty-nine such mystery cases, most of them picked up through respiratory surveillance. Part of the testing protocol from early in the pandemic was to routinely do COVID-19 tests on all patients presenting with respiratory illnesses at public health facilities, and several cases were caught this way. Any positive that was not imported, or a contact of a confirmed case, was a cause of concern, a sign that the virus had gotten out of control, that we were in community spread. We did of course get to community spread in September, but before that, the origin of every known COVID-19 case was investigated.

One of the earliest cases was a young man in Kingston, although it was never discovered how he contracted the virus. He presented with symptoms at his doctor around the second week of March, and his positive test result was returned on March 15, making him one of Jamaica's first cases. His only travel history was to Trinidad and Tobago, where he had celebrated carnival. Trinidad carnival, like the Rio Carnaval and the Mardi Gras celebration, culminates on the day before Ash Wednesday, after weeks of parties, concerts, and festivities.

In 2020, Ash Wednesday fell on February 26; the many Jamaicans who go to Trinidad Carnival usually return home on that day. It therefore seemed unlikely that he could have contracted it in Trinidad, because more than two weeks had passed since he had left up to when he presented with symptoms. Also, Trinidad did not have any known cases of COVID-19 until March 12, and that case was imported, as were the other dozen or so cases that followed.

If he had indeed caught it in Trinidad at Carnival, then Trinidad was extremely lucky that they did not have an outbreak. Trinidad took a huge risk in proceeding with Carnival in 2020, no doubt because Carnival is extremely important to the Trinidadian economy. But considering what happened in New Orleans, they were betting against high odds. New Orleans was one of the first and largest hotspots for the coronavirus in the US, with one of the highest death rates at the time. The Mardi Gras festivities were later identified as having accelerated the spread of the disease in the New Orleans area.[24] Like New Orleans, thousands of people from all over the world travel to

---

[24] "New Orleans, 'Spring Breakers' Hot Spot, Is Now a Virus Hot Spot," *The New York Times*, April 13, 2020, www.nytimes.com/2020/04/13/us/coronavirus-new-orleans-mardi-gras.html.

Trinidad for the event, and had the virus been present there, it could have led to thousands of infections throughout the Caribbean.

Then there was the mystery case at the May Pen Hospital. Like all the other public hospitals in Jamaica, it had repurposed the female surgical ward as a COVID-19 isolation ward. While the ward was being retrofitted, all COVID-19 patients and suspected cases were transferred to Mandeville Regional Hospital. When an Alorica worker (the business processing outsourcing entity [BPO] had a workplace cluster outbreak), who was supposed to have been self-quarantining, was discovered to have visited her baby on the pediatric ward, it triggered a round of testing on the ward as precautionary surveillance. There was one positive result: a two-year-old child, who, because of challenges they had been born with, had never left the hospital since birth. This is what we call in Jamaica a "social case," and it is a significant problem for public health. These are patients who have recovered from an illness but, for various reasons, do not have anywhere to go once they are discharged. That positive result then triggered a broader surveillance exercise, and over eighty healthcare workers who worked on the ward, or who might otherwise have come into contact with the child, tested negative. The BPO worker was negative. No one else working at the May Pen Hospital fell ill. We never discovered how that child contracted the virus. The child never had any symptoms, and ultimately, the hospital management questioned if the child's test result was a false positive.

Another mystery that had us on high alert was a staff member in the St. Ann Infirmary who tested positive in June. By June, we were moving towards reopening, and the MOHW began to do routine surveillance in various vulnerable populations across the island—the prisons, the infirmaries, and nursing homes. We began with the infirmaries, going to each parish, swabbing staff members and residents. Each of Jamaica's parishes has a state-funded infirmary, which is administered by the Outdoor Poor Department of the local municipality. They provide care for the poor and destitute who are unable to work or look after themselves due to mental or physical causes. One of the first restrictions enacted nationally was to disallow visits to infirmaries, precisely because the persons there were vulnerable due to their age and health, and also because with so many people in such close proximity, a contagious disease like COVID-19 would spread rapidly. Visits to children's homes, elder care facilities, and prisons had also been paused, for the same reason.

How the young man contracted it was never discovered: he lived alone, had only been going to work and back home again since the stay-at-home orders were issued, and had had no contact with anyone outside of the infirmary in several weeks. Fortunately, he was the only person who tested positive among all those tested in those facilities, throughout the entire island. In retrospect, he might have been a false positive also.

All these cases demonstrate how the tensions, fears, and uncertainties manifested in the pandemic, particularly in the first months. We couldn't have known then that we needn't have been so assiduous, that we went to such lengths for an asymptomatic outlier positive case.

No Playbook |

It's 9/11 wrapped in Zika wrapped in 2008.[25]
—Rolando Aedo

The most overused word in 2020 was *unprecedented. Unparalleled, unique, exceptional, unusual, extraordinary, rare, unheard of*—all to say the same thing: that things happened for the first time in Jamaica and everywhere else in the world. When everything changes and you are faced with a situation that you have no experience to draw on, not your own or anyone else's, it's extraordinary.

Jamaica had been through many crises in the past: devastating hurricanes, a financial sector collapse that was one of the worst in the world, a standoff between the state security forces and one powerful alleged criminal that brought the country to a standstill and led to a prime minister's resignation, and one of the highest murder rates in the world as well as decades-long economic stagnation. But this was a hurricane, a financial crisis, and a public health emergency headlined by a never-before-seen highly contagious virus all rolled into one.

Historically, while Jamaica had its own experiences with previous epidemics, there were few situations to draw from:

A cholera epidemic killed thirteen thousand people over three months in 1850 and continued for another two years, ultimately wiping out forty thousand, one-tenth of the population. In the 1950s, a polio outbreak killed ninety-four people, and there were four subsequent outbreaks over the next thirty years, but we knew what the disease was and what to do about it. Polio was eradicated in Jamaica, thanks to widespread vaccination, in 1982. Endemic measles transmission was interrupted in 1991, and rubella circulation was interrupted in

---

[25] Rolando Aedo, chief operating officer at the Greater Miami Convention & Visitors Bureau.

2000, also a result of mandatory vaccination of children. There had been influenza pandemics more recently. In 2005, we prepared for the severe acute respiratory syndrome (SARS); fortunately, it did not touch down in Jamaica. The Hong Kong flu in 1968 and the Asian flu in 1957 also affected Jamaica but were nowhere the scale of COVID-19.

The Spanish flu pandemic of 1918 was the closest in how it manifested in Jamaica and how it spread across the world. The disease spread rapidly and touched almost every part of the globe. It came in two waves. The first began in March 1918, probably in the Midwestern United States and then rapidly spread to Europe, Asia, and North Africa, reaching Australia by July. The mortality rate was relatively low. A second and more disastrous wave of infection occurred in late August 1918 and continued into 1919. This outbreak possibly originated in France from where it rapidly engulfed the world. It has been variously estimated that the pandemic killed in the region 30 million or more people worldwide, considerably more than the total casualties of the First World War. Ironically, it was the movement of people, especially soldiers, in the context of the war, that took the disease so far and wide. The 1918–19 pandemic was the most devastating infectious disease to affect the world since the Black Death ravaged much of Asia and Europe in the mid-fourteenth century.[26]

Jamaica was hit by the Spanish flu's second wave. The outbreak was sudden and severe, brought to the region by ships from North American ports and up from Central America by the banana boats. Jamaica was the first Caribbean territory (at the time that's what we were, a territory) to be affected, and the worst. The first recorded case was in October 1918; hospital admissions for influenza were up by 157 percent over the comparable period the year prior. The influenza-specific death rate in 1918 was 329 per 1,000 people, while in non-outbreak years it was 8 to 1,000. It caught the authorities unaware, and major offices of state, such as the Colonial Office, barely stirred themselves and when they did, it was in a laggardly fashion. Their

---

26 David Killingray, "A New 'Imperial Disease': The Influenza Pandemic of 1918–9 and its Impact on the British Empire," *Caribbean Quarterly*, Vol. 49, No. 4, (December 2003), 30–49.

attempts to regulate and control the illness were largely ineffective; at the same time, the medical means to deal with the infection were limited and slight. The *Gleaner* editorial of October 17, 1918, sounded so similar to what was happening in 2020:

> It has "downed" many people in Montego Bay and Port Antonio. The hospital in the latter place is full, workers in various stores and businesses are incapacitated. Some deaths have taken place and there may be more; but we are better equipped to deal with epidemics in these modern days and our expectation is that this outbreak of influenza will so be handled that it will speedily be chocked. The precautions to take against it should be as widely published as possible, and everyone in the island should follow the advice given by the medical authorities. By our thus acting promptly and sensibly, the effects of the ailment will be greatly minimised. It can and will spread all over the island: we must, rid ourselves of it as quickly as possible. Every precaution must be duly observed. If we neglect this we shall pay the bitter penalty.
>
> —The Daily *Gleaner*, editorial page, October 17, 1918

After two months of school closures, bans on public gatherings, local travel bans, disinfection of public transportation, opening of emergency hospitals and soup kitchens, and health education, by December 1918, the pandemic had waned in Jamaica, though it continued to devastate in other parts of the world.

The outlook for such a quick recovery from COVID-19 was not looking so promising. At that point, given the information in front of me, I couldn't see normalcy returning for several months, and that was contingent on so many factors, many out of our control. But I had no way of knowing. No one did. Previous pandemics and epidemics were not useful for drawing lessons. We observed what other countries were doing, sought to replicate what appeared to work, and do the opposite of what didn't. Many "learned persons" wanted us to adopt what wealthier countries were doing. Yet there wasn't a favourable example to follow. The developed world was faring pretty badly. Any response had to be tailored to Jamaica's unique particularities. And still, we had no way of knowing if what we were doing was the best decision to make. No one knew.

The most we could be sure of, from what we had seen in Italy and Spain, respectively, was that (a) one single infected person could spread the infection to dozens of others and (b) large groups of people were dangerous. When on March 27, UK Prime Minister Boris Johnson tested positive for COVID-19, that taught us that not taking the threat seriously and not taking early action could spell disaster. We also considered that the path we had embarked on—to expand the public health facilities' capacity to treat the disease with new isolation wards and equipment, while doing our utmost to curtail the spread was correct, given how so many other countries were overwhelmed by the number of ill people, with devastating results.

Dealing with the economic aspects of the pandemic, especially the fallout, was another exercise in uncharted territory. When the finance minister, the Honourable Dr. Nigel Clarke, presented an unbudgeted J$25 billion (US$160 million) package to mitigate against the expected negative impact of COVID-19 on the local economy, it was the largest fiscal stimulus in Jamaica's history. The stimulus included cash transfers to businesses in targeted sectors, to individuals who had lost their employment as a result of the COVID-19 crisis, and support for the poor and vulnerable via grants. That had never happened before.

When Seven Mile and Eight Mile in Bull Bay were quarantined for two weeks, they were the first such community quarantines Jamaica had ever known. It was done to stem the risk of community spread, given that Patient One stayed there and moved around so extensively with the large family gatherings that took place due to the grandmother's funeral.

When every public hospital on the island got a designated isolation ward—a massive infrastructure adjustment over a short space of time—that was definitely out of the ordinary.

When we closed our borders to passenger travel on March 24, 2020, for over two months, that was a unique situation.

When school was closed for weeks, and then months, and then years...

When more than 50 percent of the workforce worked from home...

When I worked eighteen-hour days alongside my team...

When streets that were normally choked at peak hours were empty...

When nightlife ceased...

When food and grocery delivery and online businesses thrived...

When it became unusual not to wear a face mask...

When at the door of every establishment your hands were sprayed with alcohol...

When people stopped shaking hands and stopped hugging each other...

All these were all unheard of before COVID-19.

These were unparalleled happenings, in my lifetime or in anyone's lifetime. A version of the sentiment: "I could really go for some precedented times right now" made light of the situation.

Mistakes were made that we only could have known in retrospect, once we had more information. But at the time, we were working with all we had, and it later turned out we were wrong. Face masks were one of those things. The advice from the WHO, which our clinicians didn't question because they didn't have evidence to base a different opinion on, was that face masks were not helpful or necessary and in fact could make transmission of the virus more likely, not less. Also, there was a shortage, and the general public using them meant there were fewer for healthcare workers, for whom they were recommended. In that first month, medical experts around the world simply did not have good evidence about how the virus spread. Once the evidence began to be generated, it became clear that masks did in fact help stem virus transmission, and by April 20, it was mandatory to wear a mask in public.

There were other more egregious mistakes. Oversights. Things that slipped through the cracks in the rush to do so many things that had never been done before, many which had never been imagined. The coordination of different government agencies and entities that had no pre-existing relationship within which to work together.

Five thousand travelers arrived in the few days before we closed the border on March 21, then left from the airport, and we hadn't taken down any information for them. Though it might have seemed like it would have been straightforward enough to do this, the Passport and Immigration Control Agency (PICA) had the passport numbers, customs had the addresses, and the airlines had the manifest. Even when we got the forms, many weren't filled out correctly.

In hindsight, we should have anticipated the rush and properly documented the people as they arrived, reconciling the flight manifest with the customs list with the PICA list. We ended up appealing to those who had come in on those flights to make themselves known to the authorities so they could be monitored. So, few presented themselves that it wasn't until the prime minister announced that people would be prosecuted if they did not come forward that we got a worthwhile response.

Other mistakes were forecasting errors. We should have spent more on increasing testing capacity at an earlier stage. We procured equipment and materials for thousands of tests a day, but we soon needed ten times that to adequately manage the testing requirements. We didn't anticipate how hesitant Jamaicans would be to take the vaccine, and by the time it became clear, there were so many things that we would have, could have, and should have done, but the moment had passed.

Despite the missteps, I never had the sense that something sinister was at work. With the exception, much later on, of apparent sabotage of the cold storage at the National Health Fund facility where vaccines were kept, there was a spirit of unity, of wanting to play a part, of endeavouring to help. There were few instances where it was clear that fecklessness, or mal-intent was at play. And that's a given for a low-trust society like Jamaica's.

For a while, there was an expectation that sooner or later we would return to what we considered normal—our everyday lives that no one could have seen would have come to an abrupt halt. But even the not knowing was brand new. No one, not in Jamaica, not anywhere else in the world, had experienced this before. The situation was incomparable to anything else.

It was, for want of a more original word, unprecedented.

Behind the Curve |

By the end of March, Jamaica held the enviable position of having the slowest rate of spread of any country in the Caribbean and the lowest per capita infection rate in the region. By that time, the progress of the disease in the US and many European countries was on such a completely different scale that there was no basis for comparison. In the hardest-hit areas, such as New York City, health systems were completely overwhelmed, and the death toll was high. By the end of March, more than a thousand people died in New York City, and New York state was the coronavirus epicenter of the world, having surpassed Hubei in China, where the virus emerged.[27] Video footage emerged of refrigerated trailer trucks parked outside hospitals to hold the COVID dead that the hospital morgue couldn't contain. This hit close, as the area is home to many Jamaicans in the diaspora, and several Jamaicans died in that surge. In mid-April, it was reported that seventy Jamaicans, mostly in New York, died of COVID-19 in the US.[28]

We were only three weeks into the pandemic, still with no understanding of the protracted pandemic ahead of us. One of Jamaica's most influential journalists Cliff Hughes released a video clip praising the government's handling of the crisis. He singled out "the triumvirate" of the prime minister; the minister of finance, Nigel Clarke; and myself, as leading the country steadfastly and admirably. I was flattered, but I was uncomfortable with the praise. I knew then that it was early days, and I felt it premature to deliver such an appraisal. I feared these words coming back to haunt us.

The preoccupation was with staving off a surge, and with "flattening the curve"—keeping transmission rate low for as long as possible—

---

[27] "Coronavirus Live Updates: Trump Says US Deaths Will Peak in Two Weeks," *CNBC*, March 31, 2020, www.cnbc.com/2020/03/31/coronavirus-latest-updates.html.
[28] "More than 70 Jamaicans dead in the US from COVID-19," April 14, 2020, Radio Jamaica Online, www.radiojamaicanewsonline.com/local/more-than-70-jamaicans-dead-in-the-us-from-covid-19.

to keep from entering a surge. A surge was inevitable, but the longer we could keep it off, the more time we had to prepare. If we were overwhelmed before we had equipped ourselves and built our hospital capacity, I was certain that our healthcare system would not manage.

In some regards, Cliff was correct: the prime minister led with the ultimate steady hand. His calm demeanour in the press conferences mirrored his handling of behind-closed-door meetings. His grasp of the gravity of the situation undergirded his ability to process reams of new information, including new technical and scientific concepts. The minister of finance from the outset was concerned about the economic and social impact of the pandemic measures and constantly calculated and recalculated the non-public health implications of the measures. He kept the economic reality of the pandemic always on the table.

But I was uncomfortable with the impression that it was us three doing all the work. While Cliff put the three of us at the forefront, it wasn't us alone in the political leadership who were going all out. Cliff couldn't see, or didn't choose to point out, that in the background, the minister of local government, Hon. Desmond McKenzie; the minister of foreign affairs and foreign trade and senator, Hon. Kamina Johnson-Smith; the minister of tourism, Hon. Edmund Bartlett; the minister of transport, Hon. Robert (Bobby) Montague; the minister of national security, Hon. Dr. Horace Chang; the state minister of national security, Hon. Matthew Samuda; and others were also all working around the clock as part of the response.

Moreover, there was another critical triumvirate working behind the scenes. Whatever part I played in what the country had managed to achieve was not my own doing, but was the product of endless hours of dialogue and wrangling, sometimes contentious, between me, the permanent secretary at the MOHW, and the chief medical officer.

The CMO of Jamaica is the most senior government advisor on all medical and public health matters in the country and has the responsibility of overseeing and ensuring all Jamaicans' health status.

When I was appointed minister of health in March 2016, there was already a sitting CMO, a psychiatrist who specialised in addiction. He had taken the position in early 2016, right before the election, with the intention of holding it for two years. Our relationship, which was never stellar to begin with, deteriorated as time went on, and my trust in him waned.

Shortly after leaving the CMO position, he declared his candidacy to be a member of Parliament for a St. Catherine constituency, representing the opposition PNP. That turned out to be short-lived: after just three months, he resigned abruptly, claiming his life had been threatened, and disappeared from public view. Around this time as well, unsuccessful attempts were made to politically discredit me with the handling of a crisis at our largest and most important hospital, Cornwall Regional Hospital. No attempt is made to link the two incidents, although I had my suspicions.

Though as minister it wasn't under my purview to choose the new CMO, I knew who the prospects were. Jacquiline Bisasor-McKenzie wasn't the obvious pick, mainly because she hadn't been at the ministry as long as other contenders, and she didn't have a long track record in public health. Some thought she didn't have enough experience. She had joined MOHW in 2014, as the director of emergency medical services, a post in which she worked extensively on infection prevention and control measures. At the time, the work was focused on preparedness for the Ebola virus, given the outbreak in West Africa. While in the post, she had completed training in public health, after which she was promoted to principal medical officer and director of emergency disaster management and special services in 2016.

From my interactions with her, I knew her to be technically sound, but what impressed me was that she took initiative. Most importantly, she was analytical, studying the issue in front of her and delivering her judgment on it calmly and confidently. She spoke clearly and authoritatively, which engendered trust. She was bold and confident, and those were qualities that I thought important. The permanent secretary at the time agreed and dealt with the pushback against her appointment. She was eventually confirmed. All of these qualities proved invaluable in the COVID-19 pandemic response, particularly in how she was able to attain and hold the public's confidence.

She had an impressive capacity for grasping every aspect, down to the most minute detail, of the massive effort that was the country's emergency response. She could account for everything from the latest science on antibody testing, to the logistics of disembarking repatriated cruise ship workers according to the parish they lived in, to keeping track of where the shipment of the medium for the testing swabs was, as it was en route to Jamaica. Up until the workplace cluster that multiplied the country's number of positive cases overnight, she knew the case history of each confirmed positive and would check on their progress. She even asked about the caregivers of one critically ill patient who had been in ICU for a long time.

Perhaps most importantly, she had the public's trust. In front of the cameras, she was unflappable and spoke authoritatively and clearly, including about complex situations, of which there were many throughout the pandemic. People considered her to have a steady hand on the wheel. Behind the scenes, that certainty was not always appreciated, and in some quarters, her steadfastness to the conservative approach to managing the pandemic was considered by some to be inflexibility.

The third member of that behind-the-scenes triumvirate was the permanent secretary (PS). The PS is the chief accounting officer and most powerful person in any government ministry. In our Westminster democracy, the PS, as guardian of accountability, can be an obstacle or a facilitator, depending on their knowledge of the process, their own motivations, and their disposition towards the minister. A good working relationship between the minister and their PS is the most important factor for advancement in one's portfolio.

When Dunstan Bryan came on board in November 2018, I was frustrated by the lack of progress of the policy agenda I had set out. I had been two and a half years in the post, and while there had been achievements, I had not put forward a single piece of legislation. New and updated legislation is the most important marker of a legacy of being a minister of government. Ministers come and go, even within the same administration, and if you haven't passed or amended any laws, there's little else that is tangible to look to as an achievement. The only legislation that was ready to go to Parliament was the repeal of the 1949 Leprosy Act, something that should have been done decades before. Other bills were in progress, such as tobacco legislation and funeral homes regulations, but the process was slow and frustrating.

Though this was his first time as a PS, having come from the Ministry of Finance and the Public Service, where he was a deputy financial secretary (the PS in the Ministry of Finance is called the financial secretary). Bryan was a career bureaucrat who had extensive experience in the public sector and knew the system as well as anyone. This is also an essential attribute of a good PS: understanding how things get done in government where it can often seem that there is a hidden code that governs things. He was confident in his abilities and ambitious.

I found he had a natural talent for putting an organizational structure on things. This was invaluable in the pandemic response, as so much of what needed to be done involved many moving parts that had to be coordinated, and if that coordination wasn't done well, no decent result could be achieved. He could envision and put in place systems comprising several moving parts, when those were essential to move forward. He managed the inter-agency and inter-ministry coordination that was key to the work that had to be done, another intricate task. And he dealt with the ongoing daily issues of the ministry, which, despite COVID-19, still had other business going on. He was a devout Catholic. At one point, he said to me that he felt God had brought the three of us—the CMO, me, and him—together at this specific time to lead public health through the crisis. While I generally am not given to divine attribution, once he said that, I often reflected on it.

To say we agreed on everything or never exchanged heated words would be untrue. That was to be expected in such a high-stakes situation, and with three type-A personalities as we all were. They were stubborn, and I was stubborn. There were difficult moments, mostly around the different stages of reopening, when the public health imperatives and interests were subsumed by the economic factors. A PS is generally not on the frontline or in the public eye, but the pandemic response required that he step into a communication role, and that did not always go well. He could get overly emotional sometimes, which was not desirable. The CMO could be intolerant, especially when non-clinicians presumed to give opinions that she felt they were not qualified to give, and she too often wore her emotions on her sleeve. More than once I said to her that she needed to work harder to manage the outward display of her thoughts, as well as to be more open to other views, that COVID-19 was more than about medicine. I am certain they have their own stories about me. I had some moments that I wish I had handled differently. We were human beings after all, plunged into a crisis, burnt out, our nerves more than frayed, and we sometimes failed to summon up our best selves.

Even with the less-than-stellar episodes, we worked well together, and no matter what happened behind closed doors, I always stood up for them, behind them, and by them. When their views as technocrats were not taken on fully by the political directorate, it was my role to ensure that their morale was upheld. It was an ongoing situation where I was the person between contesting positions, working to find a middle ground that everyone could be satisfied with. It was this role that would become the most draining for me as the crisis churned along, without an end in sight.

Small Fires |

April was when things got really tumultuous. The numbers were everything. How many new cases? How many imported, how many import-related, how many local transmission, how many not epidemiologically linked? The more imported, the better; import-related wasn't so bad; local transmission cases were troubling; not epi-linked were cause for concern. How many deaths? By April 4, we had fifty-five cases; the next day, three more, taking it to fifty-eight, mostly in Kingston and St Andrew (KSA); and Clarendon had three deaths. Most were traceable to the source, but there were a few where there was no travel history and no known contact. We were obliging people to go into quarantine in state facilities because they had been exposed and were not complying with self-quarantine instructions.

Beginning on April 1, and the point had to be made that it was NOT an April Fools' joke, an all-island curfew was imposed, from 8:00 pm each evening until 6:00 am the following day. Initially, it was to be for a week; the goal was to further control the spread of the coronavirus on the island. Unlike most of the rest of the world, Jamaica had still not implemented a full lockdown. Many businesses were operating as normally as they could, and though there was a work-from-home order, it was not being strictly policed. The world had now counted over one million infections, and one hundred thousand deaths. The US was the new epicentre of the global pandemic.

On April 7, the first Parliamentary Special Select Committee to examine the COVID-19 response was held. It was a genuine attempt to foster a bipartisan approach to the COVID-19 response. It did not suit us to politicize it, and we were keen that the PNP not do so either. This was a historic occasion, as it was the first meeting of Parliament via a remote platform. The goal was to give the opposition all the information that we had, answer any questions that they had, and get their input on the way forward.

In the midst of this were the little fires, the small crises that popped up every day.

There was the ganja in quarantine dilemma. In the middle of a coronavirus pandemic, we had to be devising policy on casual marijuana use. A set of youngsters from a vulnerable downtown Kingston community, who had been exposed to an imported case (that is what we called the positive cases that came in to the island from overseas) had been taken to a hastily put-together quarantine site in St. Thomas. While there, they were discovered to have had family bring them ganja; they were regular users. Ganja is decriminalized in Jamaica but is still illegal. The position of the doctor at the facility was that the people's marijuana should be returned to them. By our understanding of the law, we could not allow ganja in there.

We had to come up with a policy. Cigarettes are fully legal, and so the first solution proffered was to allow each person half an hour a day to separately go outside and smoke cigarettes. But how could the Ministry of Health be supplying people with an addictive and harmful substance, and facilitating its usage? That was not tenable.

The PS invited the MOHW mental health team together with National Council on Drug Abuse to come up with a position. The deliberation that followed considered that people who are in a quarantine lockdown are under extreme stress, removed from their home environment, and fearful that they will get sick. They need their coping mechanisms, in this case, ganga (marijuana). And for those who were reliant on the drug—one resident said that before everything they did, they smoked a spliff first—could denying them their fix make them aggressive and more difficult to manage? Was it the responsibility of the MOHW to be dealing with addiction problems in a quarantine situation? Finally, the solution was to classify the quarantined persons as under a doctor's care and issue them a prescription for recreational marijuana, as the law stated that it would not be a criminal offence if it was recommended by a medical practitioner.

Then there was a woman who used state quarantine as an escape from danger. She had returned from overseas to her home in a volatile community off Red Hills Road in Kingston. Scared community members who were armed, dangerous, and known violence producers didn't want her there. So she called the quarantine authorities to retrieve her, not because she was ill, but because she was scared and had no one else to call. In other communities, neighbours were calling the health authorities to come in and check everyone because someone who had recently returned from overseas was out and about and not obeying quarantine.

The landing of several dozen involuntary returning migrants, what most of us call deportees, though that term has stigma attached to it, presented a whole other set of challenges. It was the first exception to our border closure. The US government regularly sends a private plane with deportees to Jamaica. They range from convicted murderers to people who have overstayed their visa. When they land, most are free to walk away, if we find they have committed no crime in Jamaica. Despite the border closure and the global lockdown on travel, to our surprise, the US government intended to continue the regular repatriation schedule. We were powerless to refuse them entry. As Jamaican citizens, they had the constitutional right to be allowed in, pandemic or not, border closure or no border closure.

The most the US would concede to was to delay the arrival of the next scheduled batch. We used that time to make arrangements for their quarantine. Where were we going to put them for two weeks? In the process, the US committed to a grant to refurbish Fort Augusta, a historic site that was built in the eighteenth century by the British and was used as a look-out point for enemy ships entering the harbour. Up to recently, it had been used as the country's only women's prison and now stood empty. But it wouldn't be ready in time for that first set of deportees, and in the end, a hotel agreed to take them. They arrived on April 21, 2020.

Though the US had assured Jamaica that all the deportees had tested negative for COVID-19, the US had given the Guatemalan government the same assurance, yet dozens of returned Guatemalans had the virus. All forty-six who landed in Jamaica were tested, and one did return a positive result. As testament to how highly contagious the virus is, that one person transmitted it to one of the policemen monitoring them. (Both recovered without incident.) Keeping the deportees detained in Jamaica was another headache. One attempted to escape by climbing from his room balcony up on to the roof; that failed when one rooftop caved in with him.

But there were gaps, and perhaps understandably so. In a small society with a strong informal culture, a few persons of means and influence managed to make it into the island despite the border closure. Some under the radar, others not so much. Quarantining at home in their private quarters rather than in designated institutions was possible to some even before it became policy. I was often contacted directly by people seeking special privileges, people from all walks of life. But it was the more affluent oftentimes that had the greatest expectations and greatest sense of entitlement. I struggled at times to balance my obligation to my duty as the chief public health servant and the pressures from other interests who saw public health as an obstacle to personal privileges.

I was reminded that in Jamaica, money and connections can put a person above the law, where the rules don't apply to them. As distasteful as I found it, I knew that there were some cases where people came under a lot of pressure. In a country as small as Jamaica, where there are so few degrees of separation and with an election nearing, none of us could risk burning bridges with rich, powerful people. I got that. But I also felt strongly that in what was the biggest health threat to mankind and with thousands of lives at stake, health interests had to triumph.

To some, I was a celebrated advocate; to others, I was little more than a nuisance obstacle. It was a difficult time.

Midway through April, there was a sign that we were in community spread. A number of positives came in that were not part of a known cluster. A cabinet meeting was called to discuss what the response would be if we were indeed in that much more advanced stage of the virus's trajectory. It turned out that we weren't, and the cases were traced to other known cases. But such was the general trend of each day in that tumultuous month.

Those incidents were minor. Testing for the virus, however, was a major issue. Everyone wanted more testing, and they were putting pressure to bear. The ministry was following a protocol that was in keeping with WHO and international best practice standards, exactly calibrated to match Jamaica's profile. It may not have made sense to the layman, but the cabinet was convinced by the ministry's clinical team that it was suitable.

The private sector, however, wanted more testing and began advocating. A group of high-profile doctors came together to make an evidence-informed case to the ministry's technical team, arguing for more testing. Armchair epidemiologists sprang up, especially on social media, setting out why we should test more.

By April 9, despite several attempts to explain the logic of the testing protocol, which, admittedly, was highly technical and somewhat counterintuitive, the public pressure reached a breaking point. MOHW was instructed to modify the protocol in a way that would maintain accuracy but increase testing.

By April, the adrenaline rush that had been fueling me through three weeks of long days and little sleep had worn off. Up to that point, I had been going nonstop. I had gotten to a point where neither my body nor my psyche could continue in that mode. I reached a reset point, out of necessity. The work had not lessened, nor had the stress, but if this world was my new normal, a new life had to be fashioned to accommodate it. I began exercising again, which helped me to feel better, physically and mentally. I no longer felt like I was operating in crisis mode, even if the crisis itself had not actually subsided.

I now could step back and think about what was happening. I was able to reflect on what had been done and evaluate where my own core principles were located in it all. What did leadership look like in a situation such as this? How was the MOHW performing? Could we learn anything from history? What did the crisis reveal about Jamaica, about the world, about life that we had not been aware of before? In a situation of such incredible uncertainty, where fear for one's life was so intense, there were displays of partnership and altruism, and examples of self-interest and disregard for others, sometimes from the most unexpected corners.

The ministry's performance up to that point had been as well as could be expected, but it was too soon to make any worthwhile or actionable conclusion. I was pleased with the professionalism, capacity, capability, and finesse with which the public health teams on the ground were carrying out their duties. When the test for Patient One came back positive, everyone sprang into action. As often as I had lamented that our public health system was lacking in resources, the ministry was doing good work. It brought home that the greatest asset of the public health system is the people, not the infrastructure, because our people were doing good work with limited infrastructure.

I would have plenty more to think about. Things were about to get more complicated.

Stigma |

"They call us 'COVID nurse.' We can live with that. But the stigma interferes with our work. We are not able to properly treat patients. People give us the wrong addresses. They are hiding from us. There is more fear and discrimination than I have ever seen in any other disease in Jamaica."

In the first year of the pandemic, considering all the secondary effects we experienced, the issue of stigma was one of the most troubling and challenging. The public health nurses were having a rough time. As many times as it was repeated that the disease is not a death sentence, as often as it was said that eventually the majority of Jamaicans would contract it, the stigma persisted.

To the general public, people with the COVID-19 virus were carriers of pestilence, selfish for bringing unwanted disease to Jamaica's shores, dangerous for the threat they posed to others, including the disruption to people's lives and livelihoods. The people in their immediate community, who knew they had tested positive for COVID-19, more often than not, scorned them, spread rumours about them that further alienated them, and in some cases, threatened their lives. When they returned from quarantine or isolation, they were shunned by their neighbours, friends, and even their own families.

For each person who contracted it or came into the island with it, to be one of the people with a disease that brought the world to a halt, to know that you were one of the numbers who tested positive that the prime minister is reporting to a national briefing, to have journalists asking for details about who you are and how you got the disease and where did you go that you might have passed it on to others—any one of these would be devastating to a human being. This is what it was like to be a Jamaican with COVID-19 in the first part of 2020.

The stigma and discrimination were not limited to any one class of people. One of the first cases was of an affluent upper St. Andrew Jamaican, whose visiting relative had transmitted the virus to them. Despite the family's efforts to keep it a secret, once people became aware, they spread his photo, his address, and even his children's photos, warning people to keep away from them.

I talked about the woman who had travelled from overseas and who was self-quarantining, but her neighbours assumed she was sick and threatened to burn down her house. She was so terrified that she feigned illness so the authorities would come and get her, to rescue her from the impending danger.

Some were more responsible about their fears. A woman who lived in the community of Back Bush, at the foot of the Wareika Hills in eastern St. Andrew, had returned from overseas in the days just before the borders were closed, and she was not self-quarantining as she ought to have. Residents from the community reported her to the authorities: "she deh up and down…"[29] Some people thought they were experiencing symptoms. A team of public health nurses, community health aides, public health inspectors, health educators, and a medical officer (doctor) was dispatched to the area. They visited 296 homes, took temperatures, conducted interviews, and handed out informational leaflets. Anyone with symptoms was taken to a nearby clinic to be swabbed. Ultimately, none tested positive, not even the woman who was the centre of the original complaint. But there was no threat of violence.

Stigma is not an irrational reaction. Psychologists say the desire to identify and castigate those who are ill harkens to an age-old instinct to protect oneself and one's relatives from a potentially fatal disease and a belief, however unfounded, that those who get it bear some responsibility. Illness is one of the fundamental fears humans have been dealing with their entire evolution. It's not surprising people would be hostile toward someone they believe is responsible for

---

[29] Translation: "She is up and down…," i.e., she is walking around the community.

bringing illness into their community. Nor was it uniquely Jamaican. A survey in Hong Kong several years after the 2003 SARS outbreak found a small portion of the population still stigmatized those who had contracted the illness.

"Generally speaking, stigma of infections can be as devastating to the infected individuals as the diseases themselves."[30]

I wondered if we would get to the point where so many people would contract it that stigma would become redundant. After all, stigma is an attitude one has towards the "other," and that wouldn't happen when the disease affected one of your own or yourself. There would come a time when more people had contracted COVID-19 than hadn't. At that time, some people would have contracted the virus two or three times. It would be commonplace and openly spoken about. But in 2020, it carried a great deal of shame.

Some action had to be taken, some attempt made, to counter the stigma, as it was proving destructive and disruptive, affecting the livelihoods of not only those who had the virus, but their family members too, even when they had not come into contact with the ill person. We also feared that it would drive people who had the virus underground. Rather than come forward to be tested and treated, they may try to ride out the illness at home. We had seen this happen with HIV, with deadly consequences.

We pursued an anti-stigma campaign: ads, discussions about it in public fora, visiting sites where there were clusters, such as the quarantine communities. But time would really be the most effective solution to the problem. A lot of people suffered in the interim, however. Some with tragic consequences.

[30] Christine Armario, "Hidden suffering of coronavirus: Stigma, blaming, shaming," Associated Press, April 4, 2020, https://apnews.com/994c98d37d5a49c11388aba412c5e39e.

Workplace Cluster |

On the night of Monday, April 13, as the long Easter weekend was coming to an end, the CMO sent me a WhatsApp saying she needed to talk to me urgently. "Minister, there are twenty-one preliminary positives from one place. They are all from one call centre."[31] My stomach fell. This was exactly the news that I had been dreading. Up to this point, the number of positive cases was creeping up slowly, a few new positive tests each day, the curve was staying as flat as one could ever have hoped for. There was even a glimmer that maybe we had gotten it right, despite the many missteps, that this might have a happy ending.

With this turn of events, however, we had entered a new dimension of the crisis.

In any epidemic of a contagious disease, one of the most serious risks is the emergence of a super spreader. A "super spreader" is someone who will disproportionately infect a large number of people with a virus. The 2014 Ebola crisis in West Africa was accelerated by the funeral of one woman; a minimum of 365 cases of Ebola were directly attributable to that gathering. The funeral was the epicentre, the single central event sparking the largest Ebola epidemic of recent times. Up to April 14, the closest we had come to a super spreader was the man who had come home to die, our first COVID-19 death. He was the index case for nearly a dozen other people who became ill with the virus.

The setup of a business processing outsourcing operation (BPO), or call centre, is not much different from a cruise ship: people in close quarters, shared spaces, many surfaces with which people come in contact. Regardless of sanitizing and hand washing, such a setting was a petri dish of its own. In the case of the first call centre that was

---

[31] A call centre, is a type of BPO, business process outsourcing, usually they provision third party customer services.

affected and the others that followed, the investigations found that they had not been adhering to the precautionary COVID-19 rules. No matter how far apart they are sitting, that kind of setting is going to have transmission no matter what, and in the case of the first call centre, there was a 50 percent transmission rate. Ultimately, there were over two hundred positive cases among that first set of BPO workers, and several other people contracted the virus from them.

The outbreak at the first BPO, what we came to call "the workplace cluster," was the first spike in Jamaica's COVID-19 numbers. It was identified after two workers went to health facilities in St. Catherine and Clarendon to seek treatment, and the fact that both worked at the same place was recognized. This fortunate realization triggered an investigation of the call centre in Portmore, St. Catherine, where a list of 781 employees was submitted by their HR department.

On the first day of testing, sixty-five call centre workers were swabbed, with thirty-one positive tests. As testing continued, the number of positive cases grew. By Sunday, April 19, ninety-five employees tested positive, and so had four of their contacts. Of the samples tested, this was nearly 50 percent. Not all the employees had been tested; some were reluctant. We went from eight-day doubling to five-day doubling (the doubling rate represents the number of days it takes for the number of COVID-19 cases to double). In a few weeks, we would discover positive cases at other BPOs, including five at the Kingston branch of the same call centre out of a random sample of twenty-six.

The fact that the first super-spreader situation of the pandemic was at a BPO added to the stigma of the virus. Of all Jamaica's key sectors, the BPOs have the worst image among the general public. There is a widespread negative perception attached to call centre work, grounded in the perception that they are "modern-day sweatshops." Part of the sector's image problem has to do with the rigid workplace rules, which are centred on punctuality and target-based performance. It is a perception that pro-industry stakeholders—including the Government of Jamaica (GOJ)—are keen to dismantle. The GOJ's medium and long-term view is to have ongoing investment in the sector, as it had favourable growth prospects for jobs and contribution to GDP. For a BPO to be the source of so many cases, which then triggered a quarantine of the entire parish of St. Catherine, the second most populous parish on the island, compounded their negative image.

There were other factors contributing to BPOs as ideal super-spreader sites. Persons are paid based on attendance, so people will go to work even if they're sick. In some settings, there are thousands of people working in a dozen BPOs in one tech park. They are mostly young people, in their twenties, and they often form a community with BPO workers from other entities, as well as with other centres, that pertain to the company they work for, and they socialize together. There is mobility of labour between BPOs, as they compete for talent; workers move jobs from one BPO to another and form a network through which they maintain social relationships across BPOs. These mainly young people travel to and from work with each other, socialize with others, and enter into relationships with each other. All these factors enhanced the virus's spread. Family members of the infected workers began to fall ill; on April 30, a sixty-plus year old woman who lived in the same house as one of the first positive employees died. While the young people were more resilient and often asymptomatic, their older family members were susceptible.

But with the shutdown of the tourism sector and the hundreds of thousands of now-unemployed tourism workers, it was critical to keep the BPOs, as the second source of large scale employment, going. Further, the business model of the BPOs as they operate in Jamaica would not accommodate a total shutdown of the sector, given the nature of the contracts. At the time of the COVID-19 crisis, there were approximately sixty-five companies offering BPO services in Jamaica. Employment in the sector has grown rapidly, more than doubling in two years, from 17,500 in May 2017 to an estimated 38,000 people in November 2019. The sector contributes over US$400 million to the Jamaican economy.[32] The BPO sector is a high-performing segment of Jamaica's services industries, with the highest employment growth

---

[32] *Investing in Jamaica: The Investment Hub of the Caribbean*, JAMPRO, March 2021, https://dobusinessjamaica.com/wp-content/uploads/2021/03/Investing-in-Jamaica_2020.pdf.

rate of any sector in the country. The idea and the hope was that the operators would maintain strict sanitary practices, and just as they tightly control data privacy, they would similarly tightly control their workers' temperatures and respiratory symptoms.

Once the public health workers began their on-the-ground work with the BPO workers, it became clear that home quarantine was not going to work with them. Too many of them had home and community situations that were vulnerable, whether they lived in homes with many other people, or in densely populated communities, or in areas without adequate provision for sanitation. And too many of them were unable to stay inside. They were moving all about, within their homes, within their communities, and outside their communities. Their own health and safety were not so much at issue—they were almost all young people, in their twenties, and we knew by then that young people were in general not badly affected. It was their vulnerable family members and neighbours who were at risk. We took a drastic decision: move all the workplace cluster workers into state quarantine. Within just a couple of days, hotel rooms were requisitioned, and hundreds of young people were bused to the north coast. We weren't able to get all of them. Some fled to avoid quarantine and went into hiding. So the threat wasn't entirely contained.

The BPO outbreak changed the dynamic of how the virus was spreading and how the pandemic was playing out. The massive jump in numbers was startling. That we were in a pandemic with a highly contagious virus was no longer notional. It was, in fact, very real.

Up to that point, mid-April, Jamaica's approach to COVID-19 seemed relatively moderate, compared to other countries, including in the Caribbean, where people were on full lockdown—forced to stay inside, everywhere closed, the whole country at a halt. We had imposed quarantines on a few communities, where the people within were confined to their houses. There were limits on the number of people who could gather in one place, and since April 1, there had been an 8:00 pm to 6:00 am curfew. Children were home from school, and people were urged to work from home; business had slowed. But life still went on, more so than in many other places.

So, on April 15, when the prime minister paused for several seconds at the regular Jamaica House press briefing, the air was pregnant with anticipation. The nation waited. Those of us who had been in the cabinet meeting understood why he had paused, and for so long. But it was getting uncomfortable, awkward. Had he changed his mind, standing there at the lectern?

He exhaled and picked back up his prepared text. The entire parish of St. Catherine would be quarantined for two weeks, he said, to contain the spread of the virus that stemmed from the BPO outbreak. People would be confined to their homes and could not move in or out of the parish. There were to be checkpoints to control movement in and out. Quarantining an entire parish was moving into another realm of attempting to control the virus.

The reaction was swift, and it was panic. St. Catherine is Jamaica's second most-populous parish. Scores of residents got in their cars with the aim of going elsewhere. The security forces scrambled to stop them. People were warned not to harbour people who had fled the quarantine, under threat of arrest.

In retrospect, we should have had the barricades in place before we announced the quarantine. We failed to properly consider food supplies. How would households manage if there were restrictions on movement for two weeks? Particularly households which subsisted day to day? How were those who earned day to day going to feed themselves? We learned from all these missteps when subsequent community quarantines were implemented.

And there were more to come; as the pandemic now picked up momentum, we struggled to keep pace.

Ministry Cluster |

The next day, April 16, the permanent secretary (PS) woke me up with a call telling me he had checked himself into the Spanish Court Hotel to self-quarantine. His driver had fallen ill and was displaying COVID-19 symptoms. The driver had been tested, spent the night in hospital isolation, and was awaiting his results. The PS was on his way to be swabbed; he advised me to do the same.

Later that morning, the driver's test result was returned positive. The wait for my own test result became even more anxious on hearing this. The day was packed, as usual, with several meetings. I kept my distance from others as best as I could and tried to focus on being present.

At 6:30 pm, both the PS and my test results were returned: negative. The PS remained in quarantine for the full fourteen days.

I advised the prime minister and the cabinet. They were all swabbed: everyone negative. Then, with the CMO, we told the ministry staff about this development. Our offices had to be deep-cleaned, and operations were suspended. Contact tracing commenced. I sent a letter out in the late hours to staff members to inform them. Arrangements were made for all staff to be tested.

It was a difficult time. Several MOHW employees tested positive. The ministry was the second workplace cluster. Temperature checks, sanitisation, masks, social distancing—all of these precautions were already in place. There was a feeling of helplessness. It was a wake-up call not just to us but also to many others that we are all vulnerable. Some two dozen MOHW employees were afflicted with the virus. Yet working from home, for many ministry staff, was not really an option. We were at the forefront of the crisis response. We were the essential services.

The driver had not contracted the virus during the course of his work as the PS's driver, though he was in the field almost every day. Nor was the index case someone in the field; she was an administrative MOHW employee who was office-based. She had contracted the virus from her husband who had caught it at his place of worship, a mosque in Kingston. And he had been infected by visitors to the mosque, a group of travelers who would come to be known in the emergency operations centre as "our Malaysian guests."

The outbreak in the ministry was a textbook case in how the coronavirus spread throughout the world. Most incoming travelers to Jamaica are from the US and the UK. The ties between Jamaica and those countries are long and deep. Those are also our primary tourism markets, so people are constantly moving back and forth. It was to be expected that many of our first cases were imported from those countries. But just as Jamaica's connections to other parts of the world are spread far and wide, so was the importation of the virus widespread.

Among the first set of imported cases were two Malaysian Muslims. They had come to Jamaica with eight other people, from London and Dubai via Trinidad. Immediately before their trip to Jamaica, they attended a four-day religious ceremony with some 16,000 other worshippers, including 1,500 foreigners, in the outskirts of Kuala Lumpur, from February 27 to March 1. It was a super-spreader event and was the source of nearly five hundred coronavirus cases in Malaysia, some two-thirds of all of the country's cases at the time.[33]

These ten people then left the festival in their home country to make a pilgrimage to Jamaica. Five of the group eventually tested positive, as did their Jamaican driver, and several others who worshipped at that mosque contracted the virus. The MOHW employee's husband had refused to be tested, so he was not counted in the official numbers. All told, that super-spreader festival on the other side of the world would

---

[33] "Malaysia Mosque Event a Virus 'Super-Spreader' Across SE Asia," *Al Jazeera*, March 18, 2020, www.aljazeera.com/news/2020/03/malaysia-mosque-event-virus-hotspot-se-asia-200318021302367.html.

come to account for at least twenty-four cases in Jamaica. Among them were the PS's driver's elderly mother who did not get ill and had a perfect recovery.

By mid-April, all the Malaysians had recovered, discharged, and certified fit to fly. However, by this time, the borders were closed, so leaving was not an option. So now they were stranded. Their original hosts were unable to accommodate them. Having taken them into quarantine, we couldn't put them out on the street, in a country they did not know, during a pandemic. So we were stuck with them. Contact was made with the Malaysian government who eventually committed to repatriating them. Plans were made, itineraries sent.

After several promised departure dates, the Malaysians finally left Jamaica for Cuba on June 8, 2020. From there, they would make their way home.

Masks |

We learnt as we went along. As the science changed, the circumstances shifted, and new demands arose, policy decisions had to be rethought, sometimes in whole.

Early in the pandemic, the MOHW discouraged the wearing of masks. The evidence we had at the time and the position of the World Health Organization (WHO) was that they were unlikely to help stop the spread of the virus, and incorrect usage could even increase the chances of contracting it as one could self-contaminate. But as evidence accumulated that the virus spread through respiratory droplets, the guidance changed. We began to encourage masks to slow transmission. The WHO had given its opinion that people should wear masks, especially when other preventative measures, like standing six feet away from other people, were not possible. On April 21, we announced a mask mandate for Jamaica.

I had been skeptical about masks at first. I felt like it was a placebo, to give people something concrete to do, to give them a feeling like they had some control. When the government changed to a pro-mask position, I wore one because I had to, but I found them annoying, particularly because I didn't really think they had use. I noticed the head epidemiologist wore her mask meticulously, only removing it when she absolutely had to, and sanitising her hands before touching it, both to put it on and take it off. I thought: if one of the top medical scientists in Jamaica is so careful about a mask, maybe there is something to it.

By the end of June, it was incontrovertible that masks were important to mitigate the spread of COVID-19. The scientific evidence showed that a mask helped to prevent infected people from spreading respiratory droplets to others. The evidence was by then also clear that asymptomatic people could spread the disease, the "silent spreaders," and they accounted for a large portion of those who had tested positive. Masks also seemed to reduce the amount of viral particles from getting into a person's mouth and nose so that even though someone could still catch the virus, the fewer viral particles, the less impactful would be the disease.[34]

The studies showed that the thicker the mask, the better. The N-95 masks, the medical-grade ones, which protect both the wearer and others from viral particles, were in short supply. People made their own. A cottage industry sprang up overnight. Some matched their mask to their outfits. I too got on the bandwagon and used the opportunity for branding: I had masks made as campaign tokens for my constituency. An election was due, and though the pandemic had stopped the clock, it would happen soon.

Masks would be a bugbear throughout the pandemic. It might even be said they became weaponized. It was an offense to not wear one in public. Celebrities made social media posts against masks. When schools finally reopened in January 2022, the children were required to wear masks, and some parents objected. A whole slew of new experts emerged on the social side effects of mask wearing. I even had a mask incident of my own.

The pandemic in fact produced a plethora of experts. No matter the walk of life or profession, there was an abundance of new epidemiologists, virologists, and infectious disease experts. First they gave their views on testing. So much time was spent listening to others' views on testing. Then came the issuing of instructions from all corners about the role and value of a lockdown. A "lockdown" took many shapes and forms. The most common understanding was where people were required to stay in their homes, and all but essential services and businesses, such as food and medicine retailers, were closed. The premise was that since the virus was carried by humans, by restricting people's circulation, it would stem the spread of the virus.

---

[34] "Masks Become a Flashpoint Amid the Coronavirus Pandemic. What Science Says About Them," *ABC News*, July 5, 2020, https://abcnews.go.com/Health/masks-flashpoint-amid-coronavirus-pandemic-science/story?id=71520471.

Many countries had taken the extreme measure of a complete lockdown: everything closed, and people not allowed to leave their houses except for emergencies or essentials. China was the first country to implement such a policy. When it did, the rest of the world looking on said, "Well, you can do that in China, but that could never work in a Western democracy." Then Italy went into lockdown. Italians didn't leave their homes for ten weeks. Only small grocery stores were open during that time, and anyone on the street had to show a permit to the authorities. Other European countries followed with similar measures. In many countries, community spread was so extensive that it was thought to be the only option. In others, it was a preventive measure, to forestall a spread.

The MOHW technocrats favoured a full lockdown from the outset. That position was discussed at length several times between the ministry and the cabinet. The PM had his own independent medical advisors and the views of cabinet members. Again, the decision came down to balancing all the various considerations and a measurement of the risks involved; public health concerns alone did not inform the considerations. We had already closed school and issued work from home orders. There was a curfew covering most of the nighttime hours. But a total-stay-at-home restriction had not been done. A shutdown might have provided a stronger guarantee that the virus wouldn't spread, but it came with risks and costs that, ultimately, in the view of the decision makers, outweighed the potential benefits of a full lockdown. I was cynical: many of those calling for a lockdown, in the next breath, would be asking for an exemption for themselves and their businesses or interests.

Jamaica doesn't lend itself easily to a lockdown, for several reasons.

The social and economic risks were too great. The primary concern was that hundreds of thousands of Jamaicans' lives were not suited to a lockdown. We have a large, informal economy. By some estimates, half of the economy is informal. Short earning cycles and people's inability to stock up on food characterized the economic situation of hundreds of thousands of Jamaicans. Too many people relied on a daily hustle for their and their dependents' next meal. Simply put, the policy-makers understood that a lockdown meant people would be hungry. The logistics of feeding all those people would be impossible. And hungry people are angry people. Aside from the human suffering, there would be a security problem if those angry people took action. The logistics of enforcing a lockdown across the hundreds of the island's vulnerable communities were impossible.

Many business interests were against a total lockdown. The damage to their bottom line was severe, and many businesses never made it through the pandemic. Private interests and profit motives aside, the fall in aggregate demand was a concern for the country's broader economy. Aggregate demand had already fallen considerably, a total lockdown would have exacerbated that, and the country's economic decline would have hastened and deepened.

The public health risk of not going into full lockdown was also significant, but, we reasoned, once we could avoid the virus spreading to the most vulnerable, in particular the elderly population, and once the public health system could accommodate and treat a modest surge, it was a risk worth taking. By this time, we had shifted our focus from how many people contracted the virus: it was now hospitalizations and deaths that we were more concerned with preventing.

Throughout 2020, we avoided a full lockdown. Aside from the community and parish quarantines—Bull Bay, Corn Piece, St. Catherine, and the communities in St. Mary—the closest we came was an extended curfew over the long Easter weekend, from Good Friday through to Easter Monday, both public holidays. Starting on the Friday, through to the end of the day Monday, the curfew would apply from 3:00 pm to 7:00 am, meaning that people could only be out and about for seven daylight hours each day.

By the end of April, the calls for a full lockdown ceased. I never understood why that steady drumbeat suddenly went quiet. Maybe the naysayers were convinced that the partial lockdown approach was correct? Or they gave up? Meanwhile, we pressed on, still thinking this would all be over soon.

By the end of April, there were signs that people were getting worn down. I grew concerned about burnout. I began to think about what I might have done differently that could have avoided that and what could be done to mitigate the problem. A year's work had been done in three months, and everyone was feeling the strain. The COVID-19 outbreak in the MOHW brought fear, which exacerbated people's distress. Staff burnout brings real dangers: people are less focused, morale falls, mistakes are made.

A study of nurses and doctors caring for COVID-19 patients in China found that nearly three-quarters had experienced psychological distress, half reported symptoms of depression, and a third had difficulty sleeping. A preliminary study in Italy found that half of health-care workers there had symptoms of PTSD. In April, these statistics became real for those in New York's medical community after two clinicians, an emergency physician, and an emergency medical technician, died by suicide.[35]

Jamaica's frontline workers, both clinicians and technocrats, were dealing with intense stress and heavy workloads, putting them at a high risk for burnout. It was essential that we prioritize their well-being. It was important that their challenges were acknowledged and addressed and that we recognized their sacrifices and hard work. We had ensured adequate access to personal protective equipment. We would have to do more to provide support for their mental health if we were to ensure that these essential workers were able to continue their important work during these trying times.

What could be done? The structure of the staffing at the ministry and the capacity at the senior levels placed formidable constraints in the midst of a crisis. The principles of planning and rotation in order to

---

[35] "What Fighting the Coronavirus Feels Like," *The New Yorker*, July 7, 2020, www.newyorker.com/science/medical-dispatch/what-fighting-the-coronavirus-feels-like.

give staff an opportunity to step back, even in a fast-moving situation made up of many moving parts as the COVID-19 crisis was, would only be able to be applied if the staffing structure of the MOHW was overhauled and designed with such objectives in mind. There were few options. I discussed with the PS provisioning hotel rooms on the north coast for people to take a few days off. It happened, but not right away. (We did eventually launch a staff welfare programme, with hotel discounts, compulsory time off, psychosocial support, and bonus pay.)

I too was flagging, though I tried not to show it. Seven weeks, nonstop activity. I had been trying to get back into a healthful routine and had resumed my exercise programme. But waking up early to exercise every morning and then going nonstop for the next sixteen-plus hours was not amounting to a healthy balance, and I was feeling the physical and mental strain. The PS, CMO, and the other senior ministry officials did eventually take some time off. They simply had to. But I never felt I could be off the job. That was perhaps counterproductive at times, but my sense of obligation was too great. It was not logical, but it was what felt right.

If we needed any reminder that the world was upside down, on April 20, oil prices went to negative. Global aggregate demand had dropped so drastically that the oil producers were paying consumers to take the oil. The consumer price benefits of this event did not reach Jamaica because of the pricing mechanism that the state regulator employed to determine the retail price of petroleum products, but it was nevertheless another unthinkable, unprecedented thing to happen.

An even more unthinkable and unprecedented thing then happened. It was the lowest moment of the entire pandemic for me, something that would never leave my mind: the unnecessary death of Jodian Fearon.

My pre-COVID-19 schedule included at least two days outside of Kingston each week, often more, one day in the constituency, another somewhere across the island on the MOHW's business, at minimum. With the exception of several visits to Bull Bay and to Corn Piece, the communities that were quarantined, my day to day was mostly meeting after meeting—many via Zoom, some in-person in my office, and several at Jamaica House. Parliament was still having regular sessions, many of which went way into the late night. The last Friday in April, I headed out of town in a real sense for the first time since the start of the pandemic. I hoped that getting out into the field would reinvigorate my spirits and help me keep the forward momentum.

On my way out of Kingston on that Friday, a journalist messaged me and said there was a young lady who needed a hospital bed. I get several messages like that every day, and so I did what I would have usually done, which was to forward it to someone who could action the request. I didn't follow it up, which I wouldn't normally do, as there was nothing that stood out about the situation, and if there was a need for me to do something more, they would have reached out to me.

The following morning, I was in Mandeville when the CMO called. A suspected COVID-19 patient had died shortly after giving birth, she said. There was some confusion over having been turned away from several hospitals, I was told. I made the connection with the message I received the day before. I was concerned, first that someone died, then that it was a young mother. I asked about the baby; she was reportedly doing well. I asked for the number of the closest family member, her sister it turned out, and called her to express condolences. The young mother was Jodian Fearon, only twenty-thre years old.

The journalist who called me on Friday had been following the situation because Jodian's doctor had contacted him. By the time I heard about it Saturday morning, it was already a story all over social media and in traditional online media.

Jodian had booked to deliver her baby at Andrews Memorial Hospital, a private hospital in Kingston, with a well-equipped and comfortable maternity wing. Andrews had turned her away because she was suspected to have COVID-19. Andrews had declared at the beginning of the pandemic that it was not equipped to treat COVID-19, and it would not take any patients with the virus or suspected to have the virus. The public Victoria Jubilee Hospital and the University Hospital had refused to take her. She eventually delivered her baby at Spanish Town Hospital. She had then been transferred to the University Hospital's ICU and was found unresponsive that night. Later that same Saturday, the COVID-19 test results came back:

Jodian did not have the virus.

There was outrage, based on the information that was circulating on social media. Fury over her treatment and death grew, which appeared to be the result of discrimination because of her suspected COVID-19 status. But another sentiment quickly rose to the top: Jodian was treated poorly because she wasn't well connected—that if she had known the right people, she wouldn't have been rejected from any hospital. The story that was being told tapped into a latent anger about who gets preferential treatment and who doesn't in Jamaica. A strong sense of injustice rose to the fore that some people in Jamaica are treated better than others because of who they are, who they know, the colour of their skin, or the amount of money they have. "Ordinary" Jamaicans were being dealt with unfairly. This anger latched on to the horrible situation that Jodian experienced and fueled the upset. #JusticeforJodian became the rallying cry.

I immediately asked for reports from all involved. By the next day, I had enough unfiltered information to have an initial understanding of the tragic sequence of events.

Jodian, who suffered from asthma, was close to term when she visited her obstetrician on Thursday, April 23, 2020. He diagnosed her with pregnancy-induced hypertension, gave her medication to bring on labour, and instructed her to make her way to Andrews, where she had booked and paid to deliver. After she checked into Andrew's she developed a fever and a cough, which led the hospital staff to suspect she had COVID-19. Her doctor tried to have her transferred, but Victoria Jubilee could not accommodate her because their dedicated COVID-19 space was taken up. There was miscommunication with the UHWI maternity ward as to whether they could take her. Her doctor's understanding was that they could not. The UHWI ICU advised they did not handle maternity patients, but would receive her as soon as she delivered the baby.

Early on Friday morning, Jodian was still at Andrew's, in active labour, but Andrew's did not want her to deliver the baby there. The baby was in distress. It was at this point that the journalist had messaged me. Plans were made to accommodate her at Spanish Town Hospital, in the neighbouring parish of St. Catherine, which had a negative pressure isolation room available.

The baby was healthy, with good APGARs (the quick test performed on a baby at one and five minutes after birth). However, Jodian was diagnosed with heart failure, likely brought on, or at least exacerbated by, the traumatic delivery. From Spanish Town, Jodian was taken to the University Hospital. She was admitted to the ICU, into the COVID-19 ward, and treatment began. Her oxygen levels were low, but began to improve right away. That night, just as she should have started on the road to recovery, Jodian died. We later learned that she had been found unresponsive, having unplugged her own vitals, and gotten herself out of her hospital bed. The autopsy attributed her death to "atrial septal defect," a congenital fault characterised by a hole in the wall that divides the upper chambers of the heart.[36]

I could not give the public a full report, as I had said I would, because the police opened a criminal investigation into the matter. The family retained a lawyer. In October, six months after Jodian's untimely passing, the Office of the Director of Public Prosecutions ruled there was no basis for criminal charges in Jodian's death. Neither negligence nor incompetence of any doctor or any other person were found to have occurred. Rather, COVID-19 fear led to uncoordinated and indecisive efforts, and responses came too late to save her life, on the part of everyone involved.

---

[36] "Jodian Fearon's Mom Still Has Questions," Jamaica *Gleaner*, https://jamaica-gleaner.com/article/news/20200729/jodian-fearons-mom-still-has-questions.

Jodian should never have died. She should never have had to endure what she did in the twenty-four hours before she left us. It could have been avoided. I shudder at the terror she must have endured on that terrible day. Her death brought me to tears. It was the first and only time I broke down during the pandemic. For years to come, when we Jamaicans think about COVID-19 and how our lives changed and the upside down world we inhabited in 2020, we will also remember Jodian, in many ways a victim of the disease, even though she never actually had it.

Counterbalance |

My role continued to evolve. A crisis often creates new demands and challenges, leading to the emergence of new roles and responsibilities. Existing roles may be reassigned or expanded. Power dynamics and decision-making processes are likely to change, leading to shifts in roles and responsibilities. In a crisis, effective collaboration and teamwork across different groups and roles can be crucial for managing the situation and achieving desired outcomes. Communication and coordination across different groups and roles can be critical for effective crisis management and resolution.

At first, my primary job was as a member of the central team planning the public health strategy, together with the CMO and the PS. Then, acting as a bridge, taking that strategy to the PM and the cabinet subcommittee. Then, back at the ministry, I had ultimate responsibility for the implementation of whatever decision was taken. As the pandemic progressed, however, and the economic fallout loomed larger, my role transitioned to being more of a mediator between the public health team and other important stakeholders. I often found myself having to defend the public health interests to the cabinet and then defending the cabinet's concerns to the public health team. A similar dynamic unfolded between private sector stakeholders and the public health experts. That position came with a good amount of tension, but it had now become my ongoing task to calibrate that tension. I also played yet another role: apart from fulfilling my mandate as promoter of the nation's public health, I had the responsibility of ensuring that my team continued to feel heard and validated. Neither I nor the country could afford for them to be demotivate and feel as if no one was listening to them.

As time went on, it became more complicated. There were more moving parts, emerging demands, and an ever-increasing number of competing interests. Authority and influence were shifting as the different interests made their positions known. The decision around lockdowns versus curfews became more complicated as there were increasingly more variables to consider. How do you protect the population from a virus and also protect them from losing their livelihoods, education, and well-being? Public health was now faced with a dilemma. The political directorate made the decisions, which were sometimes counter to public health's priorities to control the spread of the disease. I was primarily concerned not only about the public health consequences of this shift in balance but also about my team's morale. If after all this work they felt that it was in vain, they might lose their drive.

In practical terms, it was wearying. I received hundreds of WhatsApp messages every day, dozens of phone calls, and scores of emails. For the most part, I tried to return every message and every call. I did not want to alienate people, and I thought it vital that everyone feel their view was heard. I felt it important to keep people on board. I thought I could communicate my way through. I spoke every day to the CMO and PS. I started to meet one-on-one with cabinet ministers and other key stakeholders. I took ideas and challenges to the advisory committee to discuss. At the public level, I made "COVID Conversations," a weekly press briefing where the media could directly ask questions of me and the MOHW technical team.

In this way, the COVID-19 challenge in Jamaica transitioned from a straightforward attempt to control and contain the virus to a far more complex balancing of competing interests. We had thus far effectively suppressed the virus's spread within the island, with the necessary border closures to keep the virus out and the restrictions of the movement of people that facilitated the virus's transmission chains. But that was not sustainable.

By May, the disruption to people's economic survival became too much, and the tension between lives and livelihoods began to be more sharply felt. It was more complicated than "private interests versus public concerns." Difficult decisions were to come.

After eight weeks of curfews, work from home, and a fall-off in demand for goods and services, the business sector became more vocal. They began to move their positions forward with greater urgency. From the largest players to the micro entrepreneur, the border closure, social gathering restrictions, shutdown of beaches and rivers, and curfews had paralyzed their businesses. Activities across tourism, restaurants, bars, and other retail outlets were all negatively affected.

A private sector lobby in any democracy has to be at least heard, and their views accommodated. But in a small country such as Jamaica, private sector interests can wield disproportionate amounts of power, based on their personal connections to high-ranking government officials, their previous or prospective support of the party that forms the government, or the significance of their sector to the economy.

There was a combination of a genuine desire to help the country in its anti-virus efforts, their concern about the downtime and its effect on their business, and their personal fears about contracting the virus. Whatever the ratio of each concern, they leveraged their influence. The tourism sector wanted to reopen the borders, the entertainment sector to remove curfews and restrictions on gathering, the retail sector to remove rules about opening and closing hours, the churches to increase the numbers allowed at services. Whether by contacting me directly, going to other cabinet members, or if they had a direct line to the prime minister going to him, they applied pressure. At that time, the public health interest was still paramount, not only to prevent spread of the virus, but also because many people were afraid, and we had to maintain their trust. But the more businesses suffered, the more they viewed public health as a stumbling block.

The considerations went beyond simply "private interests." The broader economy and society were affected. We were looking at an increase of unemployment and poverty levels and a decrease in government tax revenues. Business had to be given more space in which to operate to bring about a resumption of consumption, for the greater national good.

In response to this fallout there were social/financial assistance packages. Never before in Jamaica's history had anything like this been done—straight cash handouts from the government to citizens. COVID-19 Allocation of Resources for Employees (CARE) programme, which comprised temporary cash transfers to businesses in targeted sectors based on the number of workers employed, temporary cash transfer to individuals where loss of employment could be verified since March 10, and grants targeted at the most vulnerable segments of society. Though this was an important measure, it did not reach all who needed it. And it was not a sustainable solution. The economy could not endure the standstill without social unrest.

The expected plunge in remittances, fortunately, did not occur. The United States is home to a significant portion of the Caribbean diaspora. They send remittances to their families back home that support thousands of Jamaican households and provide much-needed foreign currency to the economy. With the economic fallout from the virus in the US, where job losses reached record highs, the fact that remittances were down only 2 percent compared to the same period in 2019 was a relief. It is thought that some of the stimulus money that was given out to Jamaican-Americans in the US made its way to Jamaica via remittances. However it happened, the Jamaicans in the diaspora played their part. Remittances later rebounded fully and went on to being significantly higher than the same period the previous year.

On May 11, at the now-regular weekly post-cabinet press briefing, the prime minister announced that churches would be allowed to have services and community bars would be reopened. This was going to be the first step in the reopening of the country and of the economy. It was also the beginning of public health not dominating the decision-making process. I got the sense that some of the MOHW technocrats would have preferred greater restraint and a more gradual reopening. Were we in a vacuum, they would have kept the borders closed indefinitely and maintained stay-at-home orders and curfews for the then-foreseeable future. This was the first step in "living with COVID," a journey that would be prolonged, far more than anticipated then.

We could do this because we had flattened the curve. The workplace cluster was the only instance of the infection getting out of control, and it was effectively capped and cauterized. The smaller workplace cluster—our own Ministry of Health and Wellness—was also brought under control. We had not experienced community spread. We had not had an outbreak in any care facilities for the indigent, the elderly, or children, nor in any prison or jail. The vulnerable communities throughout Jamaica where the infection could easily spread rapidly and uncontrollably—those remained unaffected. There had been an outbreak in some deprived communities in St. Mary, but an early decision to quarantine prevented the virus spreading.

The low death rate, high recovery rate, and the large proportion of asymptomatic positives suggested that Jamaica's experience of COVID-19, whether due to luck, Jamaica's climate, or to good management and decisions, had not been the catastrophe that we feared, and that had been witnessed in so many other countries. The majority of those infected did not require hospitalization. The expansion of the public health system's capacity to accommodate large numbers of COVID-19 patients had proceeded according to plan, and there were isolation beds available at all of the island's hospitals.

The next step, given the assumption that the manifestation of the disease would continue on the same trajectory, was to gradually get people back out into the world. The requirement for over-sixty-fives to stay inside their homes and for people with underlying conditions remained. The younger, healthy people, however, should get back out, on public transport, to their workplaces. They should wear a face mask, constantly wash/sanitise their hands, maintain a good distance from other people, and avoid physical contact. It wasn't about herd immunity. It was the same approach we took to dengue, for which there was no vaccine and which we were unable to eliminate completely: prevent as best as possible, mitigate the illness should it occur, provide guidelines for medical providers to treat mild cases, and treat those who are extremely sick. Just as dengue prevention relied on personal responsibility to wear mosquito repellent and empty containers with water, so would COVID-19 prevention.

We knew now that social distancing worked. The scientific evidence thus far proved that when practiced widely and consistently, social distancing could drive down the rate of growth of cases. The key was to reduce the ability of respiratory droplets to travel to other people, and so masks that could prevent that (not all masks could) were effective.[37]

Was COVID-19 going to become a virus that we would be dealing with on a long-term basis, beyond a pandemic? Jamaica knew what it meant to combat an endemic disease, as dengue had been in Jamaica for decades. (A disease is considered endemic when its presence becomes steady and/or predictable in a particular place. There is no consensus for meeting this benchmark.[38]) Could the work facing MOHW be grouped into a discrete project, perhaps for twelve months? Or beyond, even, similar to how HIV was managed? Unless a vaccine was developed and then administered to most of the world's 7.5 billion inhabitants who were not currently sick or recovered, COVID-19 would surely become endemic. Were we to do that, we would extract COVID-19 from the regular business of the rest of the MOHW. We would focus on vulnerable communities, new policies, legislation, new or additional personnel capacity, all in a parallel structure and under a project management team.

Those were musings. Making plans for the future was futile with such an unpredictable situation facing us. The pandemic, especially in the first few months, was like being in a dark, unfamiliar room, unable to see except for spotlights turning on randomly and illuminating things. The dimensions of the room are unknown, there's no way of knowing if there are other objects in the room that could cause one to stumble or even fall, and there's no sign of where the door is to get out.

In addition to the economic issues and the demands from the private sector, another external force soon pushed Jamaica towards opening: the political opposition.

---

[37] www.newyorker.com/news/q-and-a/how-to-social-distance-as-america-opens-back-up.

[38] Council on Foreign Relations, "When Will COVID-19 Become Endemic?" Council on Foreign Relations, www.cfr.org/in-brief/when-will-covid-19-become-endemic.

Politics and Public Health |

The year 2020 was an election year. The JLP had won the February 2016 election; by February 2020, we were four years in office. Constitutionally in Jamaica, a government has five years, which is the standard in Westminster systems. But the past few administrations, both JLP and PNP, had called elections closer to the four-year mark. It is the prime minister's prerogative to set the election date. Had COVID-19 not happened, an election could possibly have been called somewhere around May or June. That was the general expectation. The fact that COVID-19 happened, and that the entire country was subsumed by COVID-19, upended that assumption. It also meant that the political climate in which the pandemic occurred, and the context in which the pandemic response was situated, was competitive and acrimonious. Issues were unnecessarily politicized, constraining the government's response options, and in some instances, thwarting the response's effectiveness.

The opposition People's National Party (PNP) was internally splintered, and struggling in the polls. Their weakened leaders, having not managed to create any platforms of their own on which to campaign, needed something to oppose, and the government's management of the pandemic and pandemic-related issues became, not surprisingly, an irresistible target. We didn't expect the entire government response to go completely unchallenged, and the several doctors in the PNP would have had a relevant basis on which to evaluate the response measures. But the administration, particularly in the first several months of the pandemic, acted almost entirely based on the MOHW's technocrats' apolitical decisions and advice. The administration had confidence in them, though it was sometimes criticized as overly cautious and conservative. It would not suit the opposition to rally against medical clinicians who were making decisions based on science and not seeking political advantage. This rendered much of their criticism on issues such as testing, personal protective equipment (PPE) supplies, and hospital readiness lacking in any real substance.

Where they did make inroads and where those inroads did have public health consequences was in the politicization of the border closure. That posturing forced the reopening of the borders to be expanded and accelerated beyond the country's capacity, one of the critical turning points in losing the tight grip we had on the situation up to that point. The stranded Jamaican cruise ship workers were their first pawns.

The matter of cruise ships stood out for me as one of the first turning points in the pandemic. Everything about what happened with them— barring passengers from disembarking, the CARICOM heads of government meeting with the heads of the cruise lines—all together made it clear in those early days that this virus was going to bring about massive changes.

It was thus perhaps inevitable that cruise ships would return as another significant turning point in Jamaica's pandemic story. Several thousand Jamaicans who work on cruise ships, all around the world, were stranded and wanted to come home. So were over a hundred thousand other cruise ship workers who were also stuck at sea and wanted to go home. The cruise companies were also anxious to get these workers off their ships.

April 2, 2020, was the first indication of what would later turn out to be a critical juncture. The *Marella Discovery 2* docked at Port Royal, outside of Kingston, to refuel. Among the hundreds of crew members on board, there were forty-five Jamaicans. Ironically, just three months before, in January, that same cruise ship, which belonged to Royal Caribbean, had created history as the first to dock at the newly opened cruise port, marking the first time in decades that a cruise ship had come to Kingston. That day in April was the first time in twenty-one days that those aboard were seeing land. The Jamaicans longed to get off the ship, and to go home.

The borders were closed, so an exemption was sought for the ship to dock and the Jamaicans to disembark. The request was sent from the ship's captain to land the Jamaicans. The Jamaican health authorities proceeded to identify quarantine facilities for the forty-three who wished to disembark, so as to present the full picture to the prime minister before seeking the exemption. While arrangements were being made on the ground in Jamaica, the ship's captain, frustrated at having received no update, sent word that they were withdrawing the request to land and set sail. The ship went on to the Dominican Republic where thirty-two Dominican workers were given special permission to disembark. It then crossed the Atlantic to Portugal, which denied them docking. Finally, they set anchor in England, at a considerable distance from shore.

The distraught workers took to social media and the radio with their situation. The opposition picked up on it and grabbed the opportunity to politicize it. The sequence of events when the ship had come to Jamaica was misrepresented as the government having rejected the Jamaican crew members. The prime minister would almost certainly have allowed them to land, but the lack of communication to the ship's captain led him to think otherwise.

Just over one month later, those forty-three Jamaicans from the *Marella Discovery 2* were repatriated, the first set of stranded Jamaicans to come home. Their arrival marked the beginning of what we called "controlled re-entry." TUI, the travel company that operated the ship, arranged a charter flight that landed in Kingston on May 6. They would all be tested on arrival and go into state quarantine for two weeks. Despite having been at sea for several weeks, where they were ostensibly not exposed to the virus, six tested positive on arrival, and another six returned positive test results in follow-up testing. This was proof that the virus was maintaining itself even when people were cut off from the rest of the world.

Then another Royal Caribbean vessel, *Adventure of the Seas*, approached the island with 1,027 Jamaicans that it intended to land. They had been working on Royal Caribbean cruise ships all over the world and had all been put on one ship. Royal Caribbean was doing this with all of its workers. The cruise line had been in discussion with us about how this was going to happen. They wanted to get them off their vessels as soon as possible, sooner than we were equipped to handle so many people. Having processed the *Marella Discovery 2* returnees, the MOHW calculated it could manage 150 to 200 returnees every two weeks.

The ship proceeded towards Jamaica, though we had not reached an agreement. In the meantime, some of the cruise workers contacted local media, a few engaged an attorney, and again, the opposition seized the opportunity to turn it into a political issue, accusing the government of rejecting its own people.

This was untrue. There was never an intention to not allow the Jamaicans to land. The issue was we were not ready. As the ship drew nearer, there was a growing public awareness of the situation, much of it was led by the opposition's disinformation. Ultimately, we had no choice. The ship was going to force its way to the dock, if it had to. We had to make the necessary arrangements.

On May 19, the ship docked in Falmouth, and 1,027 Jamaicans disembarked, 200 a day, over the course of a week. They were tested and then went into state quarantine for two weeks. Despite assurances from Royal Caribbean that they were all COVID-free, 28 people tested positive for the virus. Just one week later, the *Carnival Glory* docked, on May 26. Of the 258 Jamaicans who came off that ship, 3 tested positive. Just over 300 more cruise ship workers returned to Jamaica over the next month, from three more ships; of those, 3 tested positive. In the end, of the seven sets of repatriated cruise ship workers, only one set, the 202 who arrived on the *Disney Fantasy* on May 30, had no one test positive. Again, it was clear the virus was staying alive in groups of people, even when they were isolated.

The return of the cruise ship workers had inevitable hiccups at the outset. The logistics of testing, housing, and feeding thousands of people would have been a formidable task for anyone, much less for the MOHW, which had never done anything like that before. It was chaos. There were problems with the meals, which those in quarantine broadcast on social media. If one were to rely on Facebook Live for information, it would have seemed like the entire COVID-19 response was collapsing.

I went there to see for myself what was happening. As minister, I should not have been on the ground sorting out management problems. But there was a crisis, and there were problems that needed to be solved immediately. Also, the picture being painted of the government's incompetence would damage the overall effort. Maintaining trust in the government was essential. I was always thinking about that.

The real problem was that the hotel workers refused to work because of the fear of contracting the virus, and ministry personnel were doing work for which they were not trained or suited—an untenable situation. We made a plan to offer the hotel workers a bonus to come back to work and came up with a wellness programme for people stuck in their rooms. In twenty-four hours, the timeline was filled with videos of people engaging in dance competitions on their balconies. From that point, things went smoothly.

Once the cruise ship workers were properly and comfortably landed and quarantined, the opposition then embarked on a new campaign, using one of the returning ship worker's misfortune. The leader of the opposition (at the time) posted a press release on his social media accounts, on the party's letterhead, expressing condolences on a young crew member's unfortunate miscarriage. Her family had contacted someone in the opposition party, as they wanted attention brought to what they felt was the government's negligence, which they believed caused the miscarriage. They had engaged a lawyer, with the intention of suing, and they wanted to bring the matter to the public's attention. I would not have gone about it that way, but I was not grieving a terrible loss, so I empathized with their anger and their need to deal with it by taking legal action. But I could never agree with the decision to politicize it.

The cruise ship workers were just the beginning. By the end of May, some nine thousand Jamaicans in eighty-eight countries had applied to come home. The applications were all being done through the COVID-19 app and online portal. The repatriation of the cruise ship workers spurred a greater urgency to reopen. The pressure to open the borders grew steadily, from some within the country and from the many thousands outside who wanted to get in. The fact that we had managed so many people when we said we couldn't signaled to decision-makers that we could in fact manage any amount of people.

We would soon all face predicted and unseen consequences of these decisions. There were many tradeoffs, but there was no turning back. All we could do was get ready.

Too Early |

June 1, the prime minister said, "A gradual reopening through the month of June, then full opening July 1." The 7,000 Jamaican nationals who were stranded overseas would be allowed in, in the first two weeks and then a further two weeks of controlled entry. June 1 was also to be the end of work from home except for people over sixty-five, though businesses were encouraged to allow people to work from home if they could. The private sector organizations developed back-to-work protocols. I had been operating with July 1 as the beginning of the controlled re-entry, and so was the ministry. Before the prime minister's announcement, June 1 was a whole month sooner than we were anticipating. I raised my concerns. For each one, a solution was offered. If public health had been the only priority, we still would have reopened, but far more slowly and more conservatively. The original proposal had been for a staged approach, a little at a time.

In my view, we were a victim of our own success. The MOHW had said we could manage 150 cruise ship workers every two weeks, and then 1,027 Jamaicans arrived on one day. We had contained the virus, and our numbers were low: a feeling of accomplishment had set in. I was aware that it might have been a false sense of success. The *Star* headline captured the sentiment: "Too Early to Celebrate." Nevertheless, the priorities had shifted, and the first stage of reopening the country was upon us.

The only option was to prepare and do our best to keep up with what the political directorate had decided. Prepare to test, quarantine, and monitor thousands of incoming people. The virus was going to spread no matter what we did. There would be an increase in cases, maybe even a surge. A surge would overwhelm the hospitals and staff, which would bring about its own crisis.

Thus, there was a shift, from prevention and containment to managing the spread and mitigating the virus's effects. That is, we accepted that people would catch the virus, but we focused on effectively treating those who were ill and preventing death. From this perspective, the number of positives was less important than the number of severely ill, or worse, deaths. That would be a truer marker of success in this phase. But the challenge was to get the public, who were addicted to the daily updates of numbers of positive cases, an addiction that we owned some responsibility for, to understand and accept that.

By May 27, four days ahead of reopening, we had 564 confirmed cases, and of those, nearly 50 percent had recovered. Of these, 235 were attributed to the workplace cluster (the BPO outbreak), which included employees and their contacts. Of the cruise ship workers who had returned, there were a number of positive cases, despite all that was said about them being effectively quarantined and having been stuck on the ships for so many weeks. The situation was under control.

But economics and political considerations were now paramount, with public health having to concede to those imperatives. The political calculus was now even: COVID-19 threatened people's livelihoods as much if not more than it threatened people's health. As long as the country remained closed and economic activity remained dampened, aggregate demand was suppressed, production was curtailed, and tax revenues were way, way down. After public health being the first consideration for several months and billions of dollars spent, other imperatives had moved into the top spot. The public health response was costing the country several million dollars a day—far, far more than had been allocated to the health sector in the budget. That money came from other sectors where plans including capital spending had to be cancelled or postponed.

Furthermore, an election was due. We had to think about getting re-elected, and we were mobilizing towards that. Restoring some semblance of stability to the economy was crucial to our re-election prospects, so it was doubly important that the economy take precedence. The PM didn't need me to point out that the management of the public health situation would also affect our re-election prospects, just as much as the economy, if not more. But politicians are successful when they can correctly read the mood of the people and change or modify course to stay in lockstep with them, or better, just slightly ahead. The mood was COVID-fatigue. People were feeling exhausted, cranky, worried, and consumed by a great deal of uncertainty. People were on edge as the reality of the pandemic's impact on their jobs, businesses, and livelihoods. This became more apparent with each day. Such unpredictability and so many unknowns would have an effect on anyone; this was a collective, extended situation. I heard someone liken it to being in the middle of the ocean and not seeing land anywhere, where the ocean is COVID-19 and all that the response entailed.

There was still the fear of catching the virus and getting sick.[39] But the feelings of being trapped and confined that had come with the restrictions on movement and the curfews were also bearing down. People were still concerned about keeping the virus under control, but we had actually done that, and so there was a sense of safety where that was concerned. Though it wasn't a unanimous consensus, the national mood that was informing the political decision-making was "Let's reopen... We have to reopen...cautiously perhaps, but we must reopen."

Tensions at the ministry were high. Between burnout and the pressure of meeting the demands that came with opening up, personality and philosophical conflicts rose to the fore. Again, I was in the middle. I was seen by some as moving the opening too fast, and by others as holding it back and slowing it down.

Conflicts over testing continued and were even increasing. The private sector was pressing for more and more accessible testing. They wanted to introduce rapid tests, though they were not reliable. They offered to buy the tests themselves for public use. The ministry insisted that its testing protocol was appropriate. Again, I was in between—some in the ministry seeing me as pushing unscientific testing protocols that

---

[39] "Are You Experiencing Coronavirus Quarantine Fatigue?" *Cleveland Clinic*, May 13, 2020, https://health.clevelandclinic.org/are-you-experiencing-coronavirus-quarantine-fatigue/o.

would harm the management of the pandemic, and the private sector seeing me as blocking the expansion of testing.

These are the people whose knowledge, wisdom, and advice have made Jamaica have the lowest rate of COVID-19 in the entire Caribbean. If they have brought us this far, don't you think they know what they're doing? That's what I was thinking, but I didn't say that. I attempted to mirror their concerns, make them feel heard, and promised to follow up on their suggestions and concerns, which I did.

The many meetings required, official and unofficial, were becoming onerous. Ministry officials were required to attend many of the meetings, make presentations, and respond to questions. They were often challenged by non-clinicians. It was draining and took them away from what they considered more important work. I was the focal point of their objection to constantly being called on to participate in these meetings. On the other side, I received complaints from the groups about the inaccessibility of the ministry technocrats. The pressure was building.

I was coping as best as I could. I had resumed my regular exercise programme. Getting up in the morning to exercise keeps me grounded. I found it therapeutic. I could forget about the day to day for that hour, and I was buoyed by the encouragement of the people on the street who never hesitated to call out to me. Those who were out at dawn, the bus drivers, higglers (street vendors), workmen, other joggers, "Good job," they shouted. "We like what you're doing," they said.

It kept me going. I needed it. Reopening was days away. Even though up to that point, I had still not lost hope or confidence that we were correct in our assumptions and decisions. But there were high-stakes, contending interests and risks involved in reopening the country. The internal debate over how much of the country should open, which sectors, how quickly, and in what sequence was still being contested when Jamaica began to reopen.

In addition, we weren't in a vacuum, and events outside our shores, which we could never have foreseen or predicted, intervened, and a level of complexity, some of it quite nuanced, came to contextualize that critical decision-making process. We were about to take a huge step into the unknown, where we would soon see that "balancing lives and livelihoods" was, in fact, "balancing lives, livelihoods, economic interests, and political considerations."

Black Lives Matter |

June 1, 2020, signaled several changes. The date fell neatly on a Monday. It was a convenient way to enter into the new phase of Jamaica's pandemic response. The border was open, and commercial flights could land. The repatriation of Jamaican nationals would commence. The goal was two hundred to three hundred people a day for two weeks. Each person arriving was tested at the airport. Quarantine was required for all, regardless of the test result. A tracking device was installed on each person's phone. The plan was June 1 to 14 would comprise a partial opening to allow Jamaicans to return home from abroad; June 15 to 30 would entail further opening, and anyone could apply to enter, including non-nationals and tourists. Even though those plans had been set, a number of details still needed to be decided on, and there were many points of disagreement.

The rules regarding tourist visitors were problematic from the outset. The original intention was that tourists would not be tested beyond routine airport screening and would not be required to quarantine. They could only stay at registered properties. A group of stakeholders and myself conceptualized a defined space, to be called "the resilient corridor," within which tourists could move. It covered the stretch of road from Negril through Port Antonio on the north coast and would embrace all activities within that area just along the main road. Two more would be added later: the South Coast from Milk River to Negril and the Kingston business district, essentially New Kingston, and its environs.

The point about tourists not being tested was a flashpoint. The Medical Association of Jamaica, one of two prominent doctors' groups, issued a statement that "the MAJ categorically states that it is opposed to tourists coming to our shores without mandatory testing." An unfortunate perception took hold that the tourism lobby was pressuring the government to reopen the borders to tourists, that the government was bending to their pressure, and that the tourists would bring COVID-19 to Jamaica. The decision to not test was not so much about any special privileges that the tourists were being given as it was about capacity. In any case, tourists were the least of our worries. The few tourists coming in were unlikely to have a measurable effect on the virus's spread. Most of our incoming travelers from the US were at that time Jamaicans coming home.

It was into this space that Black Lives Matter entered.

On May 25, a week before Jamaica reopened its borders, an African-American man died in the US state of Minnesota, because a white policeman, in full view of the entire public, kneeled on his neck for nearly nine minutes. The African-American man was unarmed and handcuffed. The policeman's colleagues stood by. Bystanders beseeched the policeman to release him. The man begged for his life. The man was George Floyd, and his death was recorded and viewed millions of times all around the world. In the days that followed, protests had broken out all over the US and would soon spread throughout the world.

This had nothing to do with COVID-19, nor with Jamaica. Or so we thought.

We were wrong. A chain of events brought Black Lives Matter (BLM) right to our table. It started on Thursday, May 28, late into the night. US president Donald Trump posted on Twitter, "When the looting starts, the shooting starts." The post was considered so inflammatory that Twitter obscured the offending message with the warning: "This tweet violated the Twitter rules about glorifying violence. However, Twitter has determined that it may be in the public's interest for the tweet to remain accessible." Trump's tweet was then posted on the president's official Instagram account. A high-profile Jamaican hotelier, one of the most dominant in the industry, liked the Instagram post. Someone in Jamaica noticed he had done that, screenshot it, and by Friday afternoon, it had spread like wildfire. The hotelier later unliked Trump's Instagram post, but never spoke about it, even with the maelstrom that ensued.

That seemingly tiny act of liking a post on Instagram put a lit match to the gasoline that had spread to Jamaica from the George Floyd protests in the US. The prevailing sentiment seemed to be that liking the post was seen as endorsing Trump's call for violence against people who had been oppressed to the point where they effectively had a right to loot without being shot. The Jamaican hotelier liking the post was tantamount, according to that perspective, to aligning oneself with Trump, who many Jamaicans—certainly those who took offense—considered racist. The hotelier, a white Jamaican, was one of those vociferously advocating for the reopening of the borders so that tourism could reopen, an industry which his family has huge stakes and where they had made their wealth. The reopening of the industry would come at a cost of an increased risk to the health of other Jamaicans, the vast majority of whom are black.

From the outside, it looked as if the government was bowing to pressure from tourism interests, this hotelier in particular, because he and others held the purse strings for an election campaign that was at this point just months away. This view was openly articulated by certain civil society activists, one who captured what many were thinking in a tweet: "Jamaican election financiers in the tourism sector have prevailed. Their businesses are to proceed unfettered by public health precautions." It was a dangerous and damaging impression and one which the prime minister subsequently took pains to dismiss.

Thus, it happened that Jamaica's rules for tourists to enter the islands with different rules than Jamaicans became construed not only as a race and privilege issue but also as a BLM problem. BLM, as it was being interpreted in Jamaica, brought social media's most vocal to reckon with our own deeply rooted, if not completely clearly defined, problems of racism and two of its offspring, classism and colourism. And the entire spectacle of a white Jamaican hotelier showing himself a racist by liking Donald Trump's social media post, at the same time as he is advocating for border reopening that would suit his hotel empire and harm black Jamaicans, was exhibit A.

It is difficult to draw a straight line, however, between the US's BLM issues and Jamaica's race and policing problems. Racial dynamics are different from those in the US, though Jamaica does have a race problem; no one can deny it. It is the legacy of centuries of enslavement, followed by an emancipation process where fewer than 10 percent of former enslaved people were able to secure themselves any property or assets. That 10 percent settled in "free villages" founded by various Baptist missionaries. The white plantation owners' wealth was left intact, and some even received compensation from the British government. In the nearly two centuries that have since ensued, not enough meaningful or effective attempt to rectify those historical inequities has been sustained, and though the population of white Jamaicans is now miniscule (a couple hundred people if as many as that), there is a proven, direct correlation between one's skin colour and one's education and income level.[40] It is changing, but too slowly. And Jamaica does have a policing problem, not just concerning police brutality and the rough equivalent of police shootings, what we call extrajudicial killings, but also corruption and other systemic weaknesses.

I had limited time and head space then to give the situation the deep thought it warranted. It did occur to me though that the intersection of racism and policing in the Jamaican context is not similar to the US, and so the BLM frame was misplaced. I was also of the view that the hotelier had not intended to create the impressions that now characterized him in such an unsavoury light. It was surely a misunderstanding. I was more concerned with resolving the problems that had presented themselves, which was to balance the different interests, the tourism stakeholders, the medical establishment, public health, and importantly, the people's perception of what informed the decisions we were making. That was ultimately what counted, that we continue to maintain people's trust in a time when an occurrence an ocean away could undermine it.

---

[40] Anthony A. Harriott, Balford A. Lewis, Carole J. Wilson, and Elizabeth J. Zechmeister, *The Political Culture of Democracy in Jamaica and in the Americas, 2018/19: Taking the Pulse of Democracy*, December 2020, www.vanderbilt.edu/lapop/jamaica/AB2018-19_Jamaica_Country_Report_V1_rev_W_03.25.21.pdf.

The rule for tourists was changed, and they were required to test and remain in their hotel rooms until the test result was returned. But I knew, and so did many others, that tourists carrying the virus were not the real threat. A greater danger came from us Jamaicans. The Jamaicans coming in did not observe the quarantine rules, and we were unable to enforce them. The tracking function on the Jam-COVID app turned out to be mostly ineffective.

Incoming |

My chest was tight as I set out from Kingston for Montego Bay early Monday morning, June 15. This was the day that our borders would open to non-Jamaicans, and seven flights were scheduled to land at Sangster International Airport. Five hundred and twenty-three people arrived that day, a mixture of Jamaicans returning home, non-Jamaicans coming on business of various sorts, and a few tourists. I went to Montego Bay to see for myself.

The re-entry rules were that Jamaicans and non-Jamaicans would be tested at the airport and required to quarantine for fourteen days at home. Positive cases among that group would be isolated in home or state facilities, depending on the assessment by the health authorities. Business travelers would be tested at the airport and quarantined in their hotel room until results were available. If negative, they would be able to carry out business adhering to all protocols and minimizing contact with the population while positive cases were to be isolated at their own expense. Tourists would be tested at the airport and quarantined in their hotel rooms until results were available. If they tested negative, then a "Stay in Zone" order would apply, whereby they were required to stay on the hotel property for the duration of their stay. Positive cases were to be isolated for fourteen days. The tourists had bookings at about six different north coast hotels, all in the "resilient corridor." It was the only part of the island where hotels had been allowed to open so far.

Over one hundred healthcare workers, together with about forty immigration, customs, and security personnel manned dozens of tables, tents, kiosks, and checkpoints in the arrival hall. All were suited up in personal protective equipment. There was a tense quiet as we waited for the first flight to land and the passengers to disembark. I observed. As the first person entered the hall, the action began. The process had actually started when healthcare workers boarded the plane to give the passengers instructions. As each passenger disembarked, they were directed to a hand-sanitising station, then to a temperature check station, then to a health status interview conducted by two doctors. This was where they gathered travel history, asked about underlying conditions, and discussed any respiratory-related health matters. The next station was a secondhand sanitising stop, then the dreaded swab. From there, the regular immigration process was conducted, but after immigration, before luggage could be collected, there was one more station to activate the geo-fencing tracking app on people's mobile devices. After that, they collected luggage and went through customs, as usual.

I could not be more proud of the people representing our public health system and all the other officials involved. Spirits were high among the travelers as they, not knowing what to expect, were pleasantly surprised at how organized the process was. The only hitch for the entire day had been out of our hands: one of the planes had a door that couldn't open, and the passengers were stuck on board for two hours. That one was not on us.

Getting so many travelers processed smoothly was only the first step. In another twenty-four hours, we would receive the test results and know how many brought the virus with them and then would come the work that would be involved in dealing with those.

We had done well that first day, better than could perhaps have been expected. But it was a tradeoff. We took a short-term decision that would likely have adverse medium-term effects. This was necessary as we sought to strike a balance between immediate needs and long-term consequences. This is not uncommon in crisis situations, and ideally, the tradeoff decision is made knowing the potential consequences. But that would entail having a thorough understanding of the situation, including the drivers of the crisis and the resources available to respond to it. We didn't have that. But it was imperative that we maintain public trust in how we managed the pandemic. The public's view was misguided. Though counterintuitive, testing at the airport was not helpful to manage the virus's spread. Whether we tested or not, any travelers from areas with the virus were going to bring the virus with them. That is, extensive testing was unnecessary and would be ineffective in controlling the spread. But the public felt safer with testing at the airports. We did not have the time or bandwidth to attempt to correct it right then. The most we could do was minimize the inevitable negative consequences once they presented themselves, which they would, in short order. But on that day, it looked good, and people were happy. It wasn't to last.

I woke up at 5:00 am on Friday, June 19, to go for my morning run. I glanced at my phone to see the notification: 12:01 am Dunstan Bryan (PS). Deep inhale. Midnight messages from the PS usually mean a crisis is brewing. He had sent a screenshot that, I quickly realized, detailed the positive test results for four tourists who had arrived in the island that Tuesday. Long exhale. It was a likely scenario, one that we had considered. This was a reason for the reopening to be done over several stages, over several months, not all at once. So we knew it would happen, but when it did, it still came as a surprise. Imagine someone drops something heavy from high above for you to catch. You can anticipate it landing, but when it actually reaches your arms, you have to steady yourself to keep from staggering.

The latest iteration of the Disaster Preparedness Act, June 15, 2020, had set out the details regarding tourists who tested positive: "The person shall remain in quarantine at that abode or place of residence, or at a facility designated by the Government, as may be directed by a Medical Officer (Health), until a Medical Officer (Health), or a public health officer certifies that the person has recovered from the SARS- CoV-2 (Coronavirus COVID-19)." Each tourist would have, when they applied to enter the island on the Jam-COVID app, agreed to that.

Yet, now that it had actually happened, we were back in an eight-hour cabinet subcommittee meeting. And then in another protracted meeting with the tourism interests about what to do. There were plans and protocols in place beforehand. The hotels had all agreed to a protocol whereby if a guest tested positive, they would isolate them at the hotel. But now that there were real live tourists testing positive, those protocols and agreements were found wanting.

First, there was a question of where they should go. Despite the initial agreement, GOJ was now being obligated to identify an isolation facility for them. But what facility? The remaining quarantine and isolation facilities were a student dorm at the university and a three-star hotel in Montego Bay. The Bahia Principe, a five-star hotel, which had been the main repository for the first few hundred returning nationals, was no longer receiving COVID-19 related persons, as they were preparing to open to visitors themselves. The tourism interests were concerned that the tourists be put at a "high-quality" hotel for isolation.

Then there was the question of who was to pay for it. As with any person who is ill in Jamaica, whether a citizen or a non-national, treatment for an illness is provided free of cost. COVID-19 was no different. So the obligation for that rested with the state. But that didn't sit well.

The stakes were high. Not only in terms of the health concerns—the people with whom the tourists had come into contact at the hotel, for example—but there was a reputational risk involved as well. Whatever was to be done had to be done in such a way that if it was captured on video and broadcast to the world on social media, Jamaica would not look bad. We also had to remain accountable to the Jamaican people, who would have every reason to question why taxpayers' money was being spent to look after tourists who came to Jamaica on vacation. Ultimately, we came to an agreement.

In the meantime, three of the tourists had gone into state isolation. One managed to leave the country. The ministry had not notified the airlines of who had tested positive, and the person did not disclose it. From that point, it became part of the standard operating procedure to notify the airlines. When two of the remaining three tried to leave, they were stopped. The airline had them on a no-fly list. One hotel took back their COVID-positive guests from the government facility where we had put them. It was a mess. Everyone was unhappy.

Ten days after reopening to tourists, we had eight who tested positive. That was actually a low proportion of the total number coming in, far lower than the prevalence of the virus in the US. There was no reported outbreak in the tourism sector. It was clear that tourists were not the ones bringing the virus to Jamaica and spreading it. It was the Jamaicans. And the solution wasn't more testing. It was to stop testing at the airports altogether.

Counterintuitive |

By the end of the first week of the full opening, where every single person entering the country was tested, there was no doubt it was unsustainable.

We were stretched far beyond capacity. The lab could not manage it, and a backlog was inevitable, which did happen with terrible results. The cost was enormous: we calculated that the real cost of each test was nearly J$10,000 (US$70). Thousands of tests had been conducted in one week. Besides the financial cost, the human resources that were necessary to conduct so many tests on so many people meant that we had to bring in healthcare workers from all over the island, which bore its own transportation, accommodation, and overtime costs. It also meant that their regular work was on hiatus. Health centres were understaffed, if they opened at all.

We were all of us going to have to accept that any "new normal" was going to entail risk—health risks and political risks. With an election in the offing and apart from the moral and practical imperatives of keeping Jamaicans safe and healthy, every decision made and every action taken had to be done with a political calculus. Meaning that the outcome of any and each policy and/or plan carried political implications, in a situation where there was a great deal of uncertainty about those outcomes.

For example, if the borders remained open, and we stopped testing, and there was a significant uptick in virus transmission or even a surge, that could result in an unfavourable opinion of the government, an opinion which could carry over to the election. If limits were put on entry to, say, non-nationals, especially tourists, then there would be an economic fallout to contend with, and that too could have a negative impact on our re-election prospects. Plus, the opposition party was hungry for any opportunity to one-up us. The stakes were high.

We proposed a new testing regime for the next stage in the reopening process to come into effect on July 1. For the first two weeks of July, tourists would be required to present a negative PCR (polymerase chain reaction, a rapid coronavirus test) test result taken a maximum of four days prior to arrival and would then be exempt from testing, unless they were showing symptoms suggestive of COVID-19. The "Stay in Zone" order for tourists would remain within the "resilient corridor." Those tourists who do not have a PCR test or deemed to be at high risk either based on countries visited or health assessment would be tested at the airport and quarantined in a hotel room until results were available. As before, positive cases would be isolated in approved facilities for fourteen days. Jamaicans and non-Jamaicans deemed to be at high risk based on health assessment, outside of the resilient corridor, would be required to visit a health department for a COVID-19 test and would be quarantined for fourteen days at home. Positive cases would be isolated in home or state facilities. Business travelers would be subject to a similar regime as tourists.

Jamaica was one of the first in the world, and certainly in the Caribbean, to reopen in an attempt to restore normality. But it came at a price: a set of rules, a level of detail, and an outlay of resources that made "normal" a risky and costly venture. Several countries faced similar challenges to reopening their countries and their economies while the virus was still actively spreading. We were all caught in a cycle of shifting rules as needed, ongoing assessment of what to tighten and what to ease, where to focus testing, what populations to monitor, and how to maintain people's trust and compliance. Many countries that seemed in the early days to have gotten control over the virus found themselves again battling with new clusters of cases: Japan, Germany, South Korea, Italy…from one day to the next, a place could go from "virus under control" to a crisis.

When the news broke on June 23 that the European Union was considering barring Americans from entering because of the US's poor management of the virus and the rise in cases there, it was yet another reminder that COVID-19 had really changed the world. The following day, the governor of New York announced quarantine requirements for travelers from ten US states coming into New York, New Jersey, and Connecticut.[41] What had been unthinkable—states within the US banning people from other states within the US—was happening.

We were also contending with the changes that came about because the science was advancing. It was found that the likelihood of transmitting the virus was significantly greater in the symptomatic person, though pre-symptomatic people could also be infectious. Also significant was the scientific evidence that patients whose symptoms have resolved may still test positive for the COVID-19 virus, but despite this positive test result, they are not likely to be infectious and are therefore unlikely to be able to transmit the virus to another person.

These findings informed changes in treatment protocols and an update to the discharge criteria. Up to then, the discharge criteria was two consecutive negative tests, which for some people meant being in isolation for several weeks. Now asymptomatic patients could come out of isolation fourteen days after being diagnosed as COVID-19 positive, regardless of their test result. A test would still be conducted for record keeping, but the person would be discharged regardless of the result. A follow-up with the patient would be conducted in the week after discharge.

Up to this point, we still had tabs on every person who had tested positive for COVID-19. Clearly, there were people with the virus who hadn't tested, so we had no account of them, but we continued to do contact tracing and monitor each person who we knew had the virus. For all the mistakes we had made, as long as we had the virus under control, we felt we were doing something right. But the prospect of community spread was always there.

Every day we wondered, "Are we there yet?" That day was drawing nearer.

---

[41] "New York, New Jersey and Connecticut Impose 14-Day Quarantine on Travelers From States With Surging Coronavirus Cases," *The New York Times*, June 24, 2020, www.nytimes.com/2020/06/24/nyregion/ny-coronavirus-states-quarantine.html.

Vulnerable Communities |

Jamaica's many vulnerable communities were a concern for the spread of COVID-19 from the outset. For all the progress Jamaica has made as a developing country, it still has a quarter of its population, hundreds of thousands of people, living in depressed areas, where unemployment is high and living standards are low. Many of these areas contain haphazardly constructed settlements, oftentimes on "capture land," where the homes are close together and many of the dwelling places are densely populated. Such conditions are ideal for the spread of contagious viruses and infectious illnesses.

Tivoli Gardens is one of the most well-known inner city communities in Jamaica, for a host of reasons, positive and negative. As fate would have it, Tivoli Gardens was the first vulnerable community to have a COVID-19 outbreak. A returning Jamaican had tested positive, and so had several members of his household. Given what had happened in other similar communities in the early days of the pandemic, when the threat of jungle justice loomed, the family was quietly removed from the close-knit neighbourhood to a quarantine facility. After they were safely out, the community was targeted for mass testing. At this point, another challenge arose: people were reluctant to be tested. The councillor and the member of Parliament had to be enlisted. The community's political leanings are strongly pro-government, which helped with that effort.

We hadn't even reached our testing targets in Tivoli when Norwood required an intervention. Like Tivoli, Norwood was a vulnerable community in the sense of being at a higher risk for poor health as a result of the existing social and economic barriers and the inadequacy of environmental resources. It too was plagued with high levels of violence and murder.

One of several such areas is St. James. It is characterized by poor roads, high levels of unemployment, low skill levels, and limited access to required amenities and services.[42] St. James, in the past five or so years, has become a homicide hot spot. This was in large part because it is the birthplace and centre point of lottery scamming in Jamaica, a phenomenon which has intersected with the growth and activities of violent gangs to produce virulent violence levels previously known to exist in St. Catherine and Kingston and St. Andrew.[43] There, one Jamaican returning from the US had passed the virus on to seven other people. Another hundred-plus-person team did a community survey, went house to house, did health checks, and carried out testing.

Dealing with a crisis such as an infectious disease outbreak in vulnerable communities comes with special considerations. Not only must the intervention be effective, it must also be equitable and respectful of the citizens' needs and rights. Ideally, there is community engagement in the planning and implementation of interventions so that their needs and perspectives are taken into account. Community engagement can help to build trust, increase understanding on the part of the responders, and improve the acceptance and take-up of interventions. We had to be careful that the residents' human rights were respected, including their rights to privacy and dignity. It was important that these communities not end up further stigmatized.

We had expected that some proportion of returning citizens would have the virus, which bore out. That proportion was actually lower than we predicted. The thinking and the hope, however, were that those positives would self-quarantine until they got their test results and then be isolated if the results were positive. Yet here were two cases where someone with the virus had transmitted it to several others in just a couple of days, while supposedly self-quarantining.

Tivoli and Norwood were the first vulnerable communities to experience an outbreak. There were more to come.

---

[42] "Norwood Community Profile," Social Development Commission (Jamaica), https://sdc.gov.jm/communities/norwood-summary-profile/. (No longer available online.)

[43] Caribbean Policy Research Institute, "Scamming, Gangs and Violence in Montego Bay," Kingston: CAPRI, 2019, https://capricaribbean.org/documents/scamming-gangs-and-violence-montego-bay.

COVID Stop Keep |

June 30, 2020, marked the end of phase 2 of the reopening and the eve of the next phase. I sat in Parliament, as the minister of national security, the Honourable Dr. Horace Chang, gave his sectoral debate presentation. A feature of the Westminster parliamentary system of government is the annual exercise of the budget debate. The annual budget indicates what will be done with the country's finances over the course of the next year, particularly with regard to how much money the government plans to expend on security, roads, water, housing, and other services it provides and how that spending will be financed. It is also a time when the government takes stock of its performance over the previous fiscal year, measures its progress in relation to the targets previously set, and assesses the effectiveness of its management of the country's finances.[44]

The budget debate is followed by a series of sectoral presentations from government ministers and selected opposition spokespersons. Ministers report on the work done in government departments under their portfolios and outline plans for the coming financial year. It is an important way of recording what has happened and what is planned and is perhaps the most important speech that those cabinet ministers who are also parliamentarians give in their time in office.

COVID-19 had thrown off the regular parliamentary schedule. Our first case was declared on the same day as the opening of the budget debate on March 10, 2020, so the normal schedule of sectoral presentations was disrupted, just as the entire country's business had been. Beginning in June, as the country attempted to return to some sort of normalcy, various ministers gave their sectoral presentations, though we were now way behind, with presentations still going on into July. (Normally, the sectoral debates would have been concluded in May.) The MOHW permanent secretary and I had decided we would

---

[44] "About the Budget Debate," Jamaica Information Service, undated, https://jis.gov.jm/government/budget-watch/about-the-budget-debate/.

put off my sectoral presentation as much as possible, and I was now scheduled for the second week of July. No one had the bandwidth to prepare a speech to the standard that we all held, but it was a constitutional requirement that a speech be delivered. We agreed that we didn't want to give a presentation that only discussed COVID-19, and so we were compelled to devote time and thought to it.

As much as I tried to focus on my colleagues' speeches, I couldn't help but think about the pandemic. The evening before, the prime minister had announced a raft of new measures that expanded and furthered Jamaica's reopening. But the news of the past few days was troubling. "Twelve states are pausing reopening over the surge in US coronavirus cases," CNN reported on the weekend.[45] Australia, one of the world's COVID-19 success stories up to that point, had experienced a surge in cases that stalled the reopening of state borders, undercut plans to create travel bubbles with other countries, and forced three hundred thousand people back into lockdown.[46] South Korea, another model country that successfully countered the spread of COVID-19 in the early stages without implementing extreme lockdown measures, also experienced a second wave after it opened up. The relaxed social distancing guidelines triggered several small outbreaks in situations such as one infected person going to several crowded nightclubs.[47]

Dr. Tedros Adhanom Ghebreyesus, the WHO director general, said just the day before that while the measures taken by many countries had been successful in slowing the spread of the virus, they had not completely stopped it, and some countries were experiencing a resurgence of cases as they started to reopen their economies and societies: "Although many countries have made some progress,

---

[45] "Coronavirus Updates: US Sets Another Single-Day Record for New Coronavirus Cases," CNN, June 27, 2020, https://edition.cnn.com/2020/06/27/health/us-coronavirus-saturday/index.html.

[46] "Melbourne, Australia's Coronavirus Hot Spot, Returns to Lockdown," The New York Times, July 2, 2020, www.nytimes.com/2020/07/02/world/australia/melbourne-coronavirus-outbreak.html.

[47] "South Korea Is Facing a Second Wave of Coronavirus," Vox, June 22, 2020, www.vox.com/world/2020/6/22/21299025/south-korea-second-wave-coronavirus-covid-19-pandemic.

globally the pandemic is actually speeding up; and while we all want this to be over, and we all want to get on with our lives, the hard reality is: this is not even close to being over."[48] (Imagine, in June 2020, there was even a notion that the pandemic was "over.")

We were fortunate to be among the countries in the world that had flattened the curve, while experiencing a low death rate from the virus. The decision at the outset was that a 2.5 percent positivity rate was a threshold: above that would trigger a re-tightening, such as border closure. Our positivity rate was 0.7 percent, considered low by any standard and well below the threshold. The new measures included the extension of the curfew from 10:00 pm to 11:00 pm, the extension of opening hours for markets, and allowing parks and zoos to reopen. The numbers allowed at a gathering were increased from ten to twenty.

Several things weighed on me about this next stage of reopening.

We had been doing well in keeping the virus under control and in keeping deaths low. But as happened in Australia, it was easy to lose that grip. In my view, the calculation that informed the decision of the threshold a month earlier was no longer relevant. While I understood the rationale and accepted responsibility for anything that might occur, I was uncomfortable with the increase in numbers allowed at a gathering, from ten to twenty. People were not guaranteed to respect social distancing rules or wear masks consistently, and little could be done to enforce either directive.

Then there was the fact that we were tied to the US not so much with regard to tourism as it was to the majority of returning Jamaicans were coming in from the US. The virus was virtually out of control there. Most of the eighty-two new cases we had recorded in the previous four weeks were from the US, mostly returning Jamaicans. As we had just seen, two of those cases of returning Jamaicans had

---

[48] World Health Organization, "WHO Director-General's Opening Remarks at the Media Briefing on COVID-19 - 29 June 2020," www.who.int/dg/speeches/detail/who-director-general-s-opening-remarks-at-the-media-briefing-on-covid-19---29-june-2020.

been index cases for several other cases, both in communities where a breakout could easily have happened.

What worried me most was the intention to "ramp up" to an average of twenty-two flights and 1,680 passengers per day. I was concerned not only because of the influx of people were from a place where the virus was rampant. During June, we had an average of five flights and 410 passengers per day. The personnel resources to deliver services at the airport for those 410 per day were a strain on the MOHW. The testing requirements were also set to change so that not all visitors would be tested on arrival, which would relieve some of the strain, but not all.

The public health system was overstretched, and the breaches were evident. We were seeing the manifestations of fatigue and burnout, with slower processing, longer time for test results, and a slower pace of follow up. Public health employees from the essential foot soldiers engaged in surveillance to the key decision-makers in the ministry, were approaching burnout. The public health system was unable to properly perform its other necessary non-COVID related functions.

We were no longer using risk probabilities to inform reopening, following the "risk-based management approach" that the PM had once referred to. If the objective was to reduce the population's risk of exposure to the virus while increasing the capacity of public health system to respond to those cases that did occur, we were doing neither. My concern was we would be overwhelmed. I was worried that all the gains we had made to that point would be undone, that the successes that we had enjoyed up to the end of June could be lost. The existing health infrastructure could not manage what was being demanded of it, and if it collapsed, the consequences would be terrible.

June turned to July, and the world came to the six-month mark of the COVID-19 crisis. If there was any doubt about the steps we took to control COVID-19 in Jamaica, by early July, those doubts ought to have been put to rest by the release of data that showed that Jamaica had the fewest deaths per capita than any other country in the world.

In early July, our numbers were enviable: of the 737 confirmed cases, only 14, or 1.9 percent, had been critically ill, and 11, or 1.5 percent, moderately ill. One hundred and twenty days after the first COVID-19 case was confirmed, Jamaica had a mortality rate of 1.4 percent, compared to the international rate of between 3 and 4 percent. And we registered an 80 percent recovery rate, a hospitalisation rate of less than 1 percent, and a reproductive rate of less than one.

The pandemic was not over, nor had the virus gone away, but I felt satisfied that the decisions we had taken were the right ones, particularly as regards the public health-economic tradeoff. The public largely agreed. A Bill Johnson poll had found that I had a 79 percent approval rating, the highest of any health minister ever. I believe much of that was linked to the pandemic management. There were nevertheless ongoing problems that had to be dealt with. A shortage of medical masks came about in large part because the US had ordered that no personal protective gear be allowed to leave the country, and our regular suppliers were in the US. These crises became so regular that they lost their currency to qualify as a crisis.

The pace of opening in Jamaica had accelerated to the point where the general mood was "COVID stop keep" (COVID was over). People's tolerance for rules had weakened. In the beginning, people were more obedient as they were fearful, but people were now less afraid and didn't think they were in danger. The virus wasn't widespread (yet!), and the death rate had been unexpectedly low. Again, our own success was making the situation more difficult to control. Across the island, many people were not wearing masks or maintaining physical distancing. Videos circulated on social media of mask-less people crowded together in party situations. Large funerals, including nine nights and repasts, had resumed, with relatives flying in from overseas to attend.

The incoming funeral attendees were a particular problem. Visitors were not allowed to attend funerals, and they attested to this on their application. Most of them were Jamaican nationals who lived overseas, mainly in the US. They were lying on their applications to enter the island, as they were not stating the true reason for their visit. Then they were defying the quarantine orders. Over a two-week period, late June going into early July, we had several cases of nationals coming in for funerals, defying the quarantine orders, returning a positive test, and leaving the island before the test result was recorded and actioned.

Among the unusual situations that the pandemic brought about was one where undercover policemen attended a funeral in an attempt to capture a man who had tested positive and was actively evading the authorities. He had declared on his application that he was not coming for a funeral. We learned of the funeral inadvertently. The operation was successful: he was spotted at the repast, where he was fully involved in the proceedings. He was detained by police in the midst of great commotion, in particular, protests from his mother, and taken to St. Joseph's Hospital.

In the public health system, the "COVID stop keep" attitude was also bringing challenges. People had resumed seeking medical attention for non-COVID-19 ailments. There had been a dip in the numbers of patients seeking medical help in the first few months of the pandemic, but now people were back at the health centres, and they were there in numbers. Crowds of people were rowdy and not maintaining social/physical distancing. At Annotto Bay Hospital, twice in one day, the police had to be called in.

Meanwhile, the virus continued to spread in the US, with little respite. The peak in several US cities at the beginning of April had subsided, but we were now witnessing the spread of the virus to the rest of the country, at the same time as most of the country, suffering from lockdown fatigue, tired of social distancing, and fed up with mask wearing, was opening up. Most of our travelers, whether tourists, business people, or returning Jamaicans, were coming from the US, and more and more of them were arriving every day. The prospects for containment in the US were unlikely, given the rapidity and magnitude of the virus's spread.[49] The course of the virus in the

---

49 "Coronavirus Cases Are Surging Across the U.S. Here's What We Know," *The New York Times*, July 2, 2020, www.nytimes.com/interactive/2020/07/02/us/coronavirus-cases-increase.html.

US would affect Jamaica. It was inevitable that we would be affected. The only question was how badly.

I eventually made my sectoral presentation on July 7, 2020. The theme was "Public Investment in Public Health: Every ONE Counts." It was an opportunity to put down on record, in one place, all that had transpired in the previous four months. The world had turned upside down, Jamaica with it, and public health was at the centre of the effort to restore stability and certainty. I recounted the infrastructure improvements that had been undertaken and the work of other ministries related to the pandemic. I tabled the monies that had been spent and acknowledged the work of the international partners in the effort. I made it a point to mention the ministry's work that wasn't pandemic-centred. Clearly, the business of the day was the pandemic, and much of the ministry's other work had been sidelined, but I refused to allow the pandemic to be the only thing I talked about. It was my own personal effort to resist the pandemic from taking us over completely.

One week later, a whole other tidal wave inundated me, one that I had not seen coming.

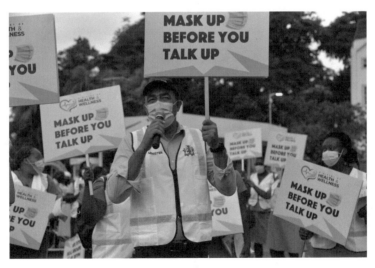

Hon. Dr. Christopher Tufton, Jamaica's minister of health and wellness, leads a team of healthcare workers at the "Mask Up Before You Talk Up" campaign launch, hosted in Port Antonio, Portland, Jamaica on December 3, 2020. Photograph courtesy of the Jamaica Information Service.

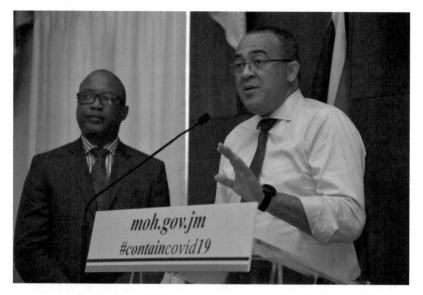

Hon. Dr. Christopher Tufton (right), Jamaica's minister of health and wellness, with Mr. Dunstan E. Bryan, permanent secretary in the Ministry of Health and Wellness as they provide Jamaicans with an update on COVID-19 during a press conference hosted at the Banquet Hall of the Office of the Prime Minister on March 17, 2020. **Photograph courtesy of the Jamaica Information Service.**

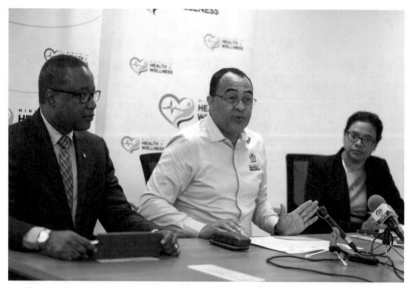

Hon. Dr. Christopher Tufton with Mr. Dunstan E. Bryan, the permanent secretary in the Ministry of Health and Wellness; and Dr. Jacquiline Bisasor-McKenzie, the chief medical officer, as they update Jamaicans on the novel coronavirus during a press conference hosted at the offices of the Ministry of Health and Wellness, 10-16 Grenada Way, on February 5, 2020. Photograph courtesy of the Jamaica Information Service.

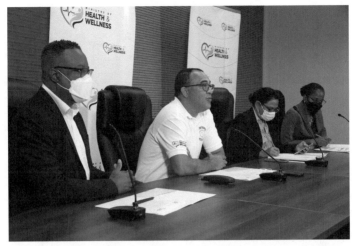

Jamaica's minister of health and wellness, the Hon. Dr. Christopher Tufton (second from left) with the permanent secretary, Mr. Dunstan E. Bryan (from left); the chief medical officer, Dr. Jacquiline Bisasor-McKenzie; and the national epidemiologist, Dr. Karen Webster-Kerr during a press conference on April 14, 2021. Photograph courtesy of the Jamaica Information Service.

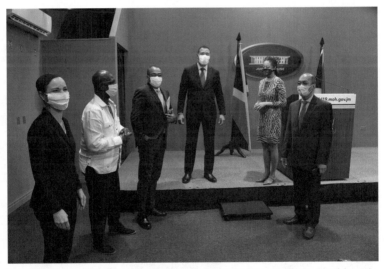

Jamaica's minister of health and wellness, the Hon. Dr. Christopher Tufton (third from the right) together with the prime minister, the Most Hon. Andrew Holness (third from right), and the other cabinet ministers: Atty. Gen. Marlene Malahoo Forte (second from right); Hon. Dr. Horace Chang, the deputy minister and minister of national security (first right); Hon. Desmond McKenzie, the minister of local government and rural development (immediate left of me); Hon. Kamina Johnson Smith, the minister of foreign affairs and foreign trade (extreme left). The occasion was the April 20, 2020 press conference hosted at the Office of the Prime Minister. Photograph courtesy of the Jamaica Information Service.

145

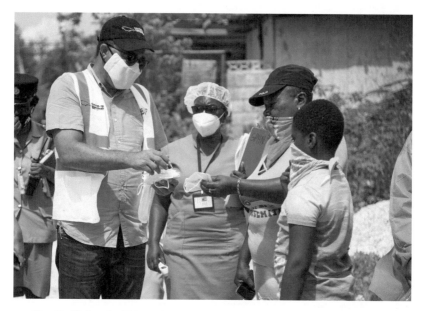

Hon. Dr. Christopher Tufton takes a tour of the quarantined community of Sandy Bay, Clarendon on August 7, 2020. Photograph courtesy of the Jamaica Information Service.

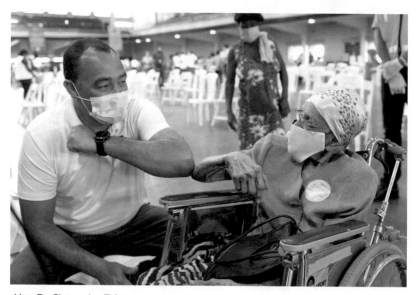

Hon. Dr. Christopher Tufton greets a senior citizen who visited the National Vaccination Blitz site at the National Arena on April 3, 2021 to receive her COVID-19 vaccine. Photograph courtesy of the Jamaica Information Service.

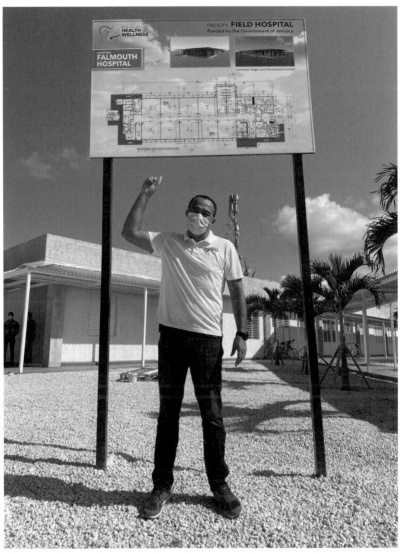

Hon. Dr. Christopher Tufton, the minister of health and wellness, at the unveiling of signage for the establishment of the field hospital in Falmouth.

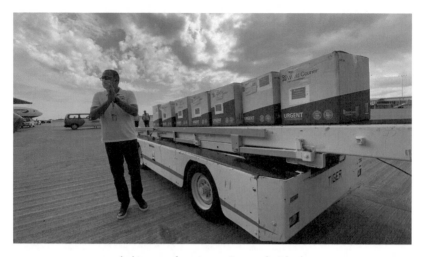

A shipment of vaccines arrives on the island.

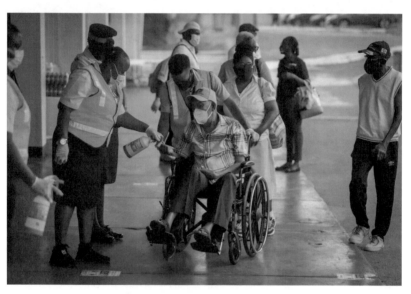

Jamaicans visit a vaccination blitz site.

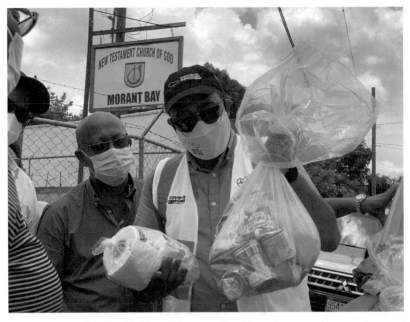

The distribution of food and other supplies to communities under quarantine was a feature of the national COVID-19 response.

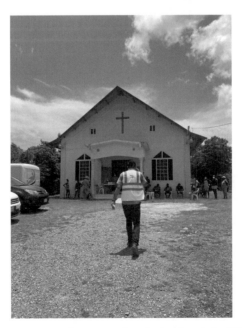

Churches were among the converted vaccination sites during COVID-19.

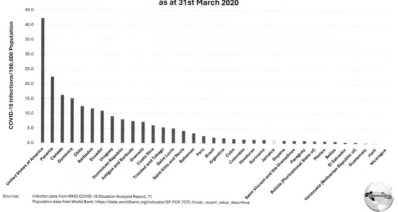

COVID-19 Infection Rate (Per 100,000 Population) for Countries in the Americas as at 31st March 2020

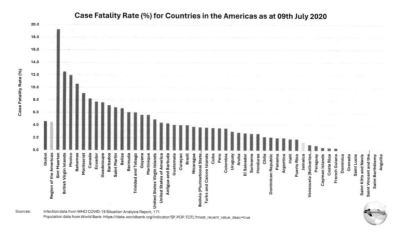

Case Fatality Rate (%) for Countries in the Americas as at 09th July 2020

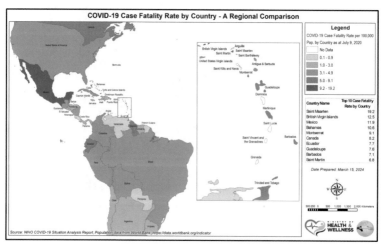

COVID-19 Case Fatality Rate by Country - A Regional Comparison

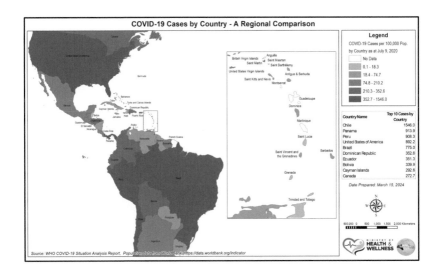

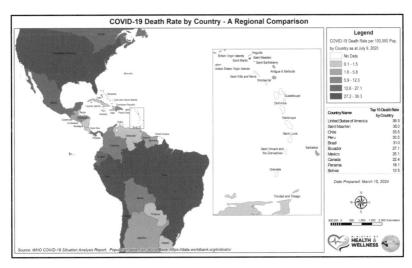

The Private Lives
of Public Men

A general election loomed. Had the pandemic not happened, we probably would have had an election in May or June already. Trinidad and Tobago announced in July that they would hold theirs in early August, increasing the anticipation that we would hold ours, as well as providing a test case for a pandemic election in the Caribbean. An approaching election meant political mischief, and with my high approval ratings, I was an obvious target. My personal life became the subject of public scrutiny. A set of damaging and defamatory social media posts emerged. COVID press conferences were taken over by inappropriate questions about my marriage.

At the centre of debacle was the Jamaica Moves Wellness Initiative. It had become a hallmark of my stewardship as minister of health and wellness. Jamaica Moves was a campaign to get Jamaicans to exercise, eat a balanced diet, and know their health status and encourage lifestyle change to combat non-communicable diseases (NCDs). NCDs are the primary cause of morbidity and mortality in Jamaica. Upon being appointed minister of health and familiarizing myself with the portfolio, I quickly concluded that NCDs, which are lifestyle diseases, posed the primary health threat, and behavioural change at the individual level was the most important measure to be taken to improve public health. I myself had been on a lifestyle change and wellness journey for the previous few years, and so brought my personal experience to this conviction. In my mid-forties, I took up running, cycling, and swimming and discovered a new lease on life.

An independent marketing firm, Market Me, came up with the creative concept for what became Jamaica Moves. I had worked with Market Me and its principal when I was at the Caribbean Policy Research Institute (CAPRI), and she had previously done campaign work for the JLP, including in my constituency. She was also a good friend. The Market Me team made a presentation proposing a lifestyle and wellness campaign to unit heads at the ministry, and they expressed satisfaction with the concept. From there, the normal procurement process was followed, and Market Me became the external agency operationalizing the concept and its activities, which included public events around the island and an advertising and messaging campaign. Though it was too early to prove the impact in terms of actual behaviour change, it was clear that the programme was successful in its extensive reach, brand recognition, and engagement. The success of Jamaica Moves placed Market Me in a position to be asked by other public health agencies to undertake public relations and marketing work, and given their growing familiarity with the Ministry and its procurement processes, particularly with small contracts that did not have to go to tender, they soon became one of the ministry's "go-to" external marketing firms. The fact that they did good work was most important, as was the fact that they delivered value for money. Aside from the ministry and public health agencies, Market Me had a separate client base of large private sector entities, and they conducted several other successful marketing and PR campaigns.

Jamaica is a small country. One of the challenges many of us in the public sphere, and too in business, face is how we determine what is a conflict of interest as we balance how we leverage personal and social relationships with the limited pool of expertise and capacity. In a place like Jamaica, a broad definition of conflict of interest would implicate everyone. Market Me worked for the ministry, and by extension for me, as a result of a procurement process that I had no say in, and according to a transparent and meticulous public sector contractual process. At no point did my friendship with the leader at Market Me have any influence on any of the contracts the company got from the ministry or from any other public health agency.

A mischief maker (or makers) had begun to send around WhatsApp messages about our personal relationship. Those were followed by a newly created Instagram account that posted a series of embarrassing allegations. A lewd pornographic video was circulated that was purported to be me, which it wasn't. Both were reported to the Jamaica Constabulary Force (police) cybercrimes unit and taken down. It was an embarrassment to my family, Market Me, and to the ministry.

Mainstream media further sensationalized the situation. The Jamaica *Gleaner* newspaper published a photo cropped from a group photo to give the impression that it was a photo of me and the person in question. The disappointment in the newspaper using that particular photo was that it was taken on the occasion of seeing off a little boy, Kenrick who was on his way to get life-saving surgery in Canada. We were in Adam Stewart's private jet that he had allowed to be used for this mission. (Adam Stewart is one of Jamaica's leading hoteliers.) A huge fundraising effort had been undertaken for his surgery. It was hurtful that a photo commemorating such a positive and altruistic event was used to malign and scandalize me, and to target and defame her. It was wrong.

The Public Accounts and Appropriations Committee (PAAC), a parliamentary oversight committee, called on the ministry to answer questions. The PS came off his holiday to attend the meetings. The PS said categorically at the PAAC, and on several other occasions, that nothing untoward or improper had occurred at any point in relation to contracts involving Market Me. Permanent secretaries are not loyal to the politically appointed minister. Formal investigations were initiated, but nothing came of them (up to the point of this writing). There was nothing there.

This was a difficult period, as it put me in the unenviable position of being torn between my loyalty to my family, my professional responsibilities, and my obligation to defend the Market Me team, which had been sincere in its contribution and did not deserve the damage to personal and professional reputations. It was made even more difficult because of where it came in the political cycle and the political attempts to exploit these private matters.

One of the difficult decisions I made was to be silent on the matter. I felt at the time that the more I said, the more the matter would be spun and would remain in the spotlight. Anything I said, I thought, would be interpreted to give fodder to the mischief.

Aside from the hurt and embarrassment to my family and loved ones, my main concern about this unnecessary scandal-mongering was that it would distract and undermine the COVID-19 strategy, that it would undermine the trust that the public had in me as one of the key managers of the pandemic response, and that if I were to lose credibility, the response would also lose credibility. Politically, it would not—and did not—affect me. My constituents in West Central St. Catherine gave no negative feedback. In fact, poll results showed that support for me in the constituency had almost doubled. They were unbothered by the noise, apparently, and my service to them was not affected. I went on to win back my seat in the next election with twice the margin of the previous election.

Whatever my private life might or might not have been, I was confident in the work I had done as minister, not only in COVID, but also for the three years up to that point. My flagship programme, Jamaica Moves, was one of the most visible and successful government marketing programmes ever. Jamaica Moves saved many lives as it motivated Jamaicans to exercise, eat healthier, get regular health checks, and take their medication. I will never forget a vendor in Mandeville Market who attended a Jamaica Moves event and got her blood pressure checked at one of the booths. Her blood pressure was so high that she was on the verge of a stroke. She went straight to hospital. She didn't know she was unwell; her life was saved because she found out at that event. There was tremendous potential for the programme to be institutionalized and scaled. It was possible the scandal would lay the brand and the programme to rest. But the political cycle usually does not support the continuity of programmes across administrations, and even though it was endorsed by the opposition, it would not have likely lasted beyond my time in office in any case. It is one of the disappointments of public office and indicative of the lack of maturity in our political culture.

I was carrying a lot, ongoing COVID-19 management, the tension between the opening up of the economy and keeping people safe from the virus, reconciling the various interests that were lobbying me every day for their needs and their demands to be met, gearing up for an election, my efforts to protect my family and loved ones, and my own regret at what had happened.

Buckling under pressure was not an option. "Now is not the time for self-pity," said one newspaper editorial. I agreed. The editorial spoke to me directly: "If you fail, we all fail."

Every One Counts |

By August, we were, for better or worse, "living with COVID." But that could only be done if every single person was accountable for themselves. Ironically, the mantra I had been promoting around wellness and Jamaica Moves was "taking responsibility," and here it was, each person taking responsibility for masking up, social distancing, not going out unless necessary, and maintaining good hand hygiene. "Everyone counts," which had been the theme of my sectoral presentation, was the new slogan we were pushing, implying that each person could make a difference. The system had proven it could do its part. We now had over three hundred beds, eighty ventilators, over one thousand community health aides, and over one hundred new doctors about to come on board. We had created protocols for every conceivable activity of daily life. If people played their part and we as government continued to manage, the only thing left was a vaccine. And for that we had to wait on the science.

Since March, we had been bracing for a surge. Up to now, it hadn't happened, and we thought we had somehow been spared. Whether by luck or because we happened to do an amazing job, we harboured an illusion that Jamaica was going to be the world's exception, where we had flattened the curve and would live happily ever after. On August 11, 2020, in a special sitting of Parliament, which should have been on recess, the prime minister named the election date for September 3, 2020. That day, the eleventh, the numbers of positives suggested an uptick, but it was not clear then that we were heading for a surge, nor that the surge was already in train. We had thought we were firmly in "new normal" territory. Getting a new mandate, which we felt fairly confident about, would provide the political space to enact the policies necessary to stabilize the country in that new normal and begin recovery efforts for the economy and the country as a whole.

The nineteenth of August was the first clear indication that the situation was changing. Up to the day before, new positive cases ranged from five to thirty each day and were usually in the teens. On August 19, we had forty-six new positives, a record high. The next day, it was ninety-eight. Just when we thought we were on our way back to normalcy and an election had been called, the virus took a turn that destabilized everything.

What happened? Two main factors: Jamaicans coming in from the US brought the virus with them, did not obey the quarantine orders, and spread it, and second, the holiday period of the first week of August.

Emblematic of the first phenomenon was two outbreaks leading to community quarantines, both involving churches, one in Sandy Bay, Clarendon, and the other in St. Thomas. In one instance, the church's pastor returned from the US, held services where he preached, infected the co-pastor and congregants in one church in one community, then went to a nearby community and infected another set of people at a church convention, fifteen people in total. In St. Thomas, a sick person went to church, and the prayer warriors gathered around and prayed for him. His illness was COVID-19, and he passed the virus on to them.

The emancipation and independence day celebrations were the second reason. Assuming that we were out of the danger zone, and counting on people to be responsible, the prime minister had eased gathering restrictions so that people could enjoy the holidays. There was also the factor that, having opened to tourism, local attractions had to be opened to Jamaicans. It would have been untenable that foreigners could come and enjoy our beaches and rivers and Jamaicans not be allowed. That week of celebration was the likely source of several new clusters, as positive cases increased just two weeks later.

By this time, the science was conclusive: droplet transmission was how the virus was being transmitted. Droplet transmission occurs when larger respiratory droplets are expelled from an infected person when they cough, sneeze, talk (or sing), or breathe. These droplets can travel a short distance, up to about six feet, and they can infect others if they come into direct contact with the mouth, nose, or eyes of another person. Transmission could also vary depending on the setting, whether indoors or outdoors, the number of people present, and the type of activity through which the droplets are being released. Further, while any infected person is a potential vector, super-spreading events—as in nursing homes, meatpacking plants, churches, and bars—were major drivers of the virus's spread.[1] The conditions for increased spread were, based on this, ideal in Jamaica.

Jamaica was not alone in experiencing a spike. Many other countries, including our Caribbean neighbours, who had flattened the curve, were experiencing surges. The specifics for each was somewhat different, but at the root of it was returning nationals or incoming travelers who brought the virus with them and hadn't obeyed quarantine orders. We knew from when the cruise ship workers returned that quarantines, when strictly obeyed/enforced, were effective. None of those who had the virus transmitted it to anyone else.

Trinidad was a case in point. They had only 1 positive case in the entire month of May and only 13 in June, many of whom were returning nationals, and who were characterised as imported cases. That trend continued into July, when lockdown restrictions were eased. At the beginning of July, the PM set the election date for August 10. Prime Minister Rowley had taken office in September 2015 and was almost up against his five-year limit, though presumably the T & T constitution allows for an extension of some months in the case of an emergency, which the pandemic could certainly qualify as. On July 21, a positive case that was not imported was reported. But the numbers continued to be low, with a total of thirty-nine for the month of July. But then, in the first week of August, fifty-six positives were reported. On August 8, in one day, there were fifty positives. Between July 21 and August 21, Trinidad confirmed 727 new COVID-19 cases. After the election, community spread was declared and T & T went back into full lockdown. All in-house restaurant dining and bars, beaches and rivers, places of worship, fitness centers/gyms, waterparks, casinos, and movie theatres were ordered closed for twenty-eight days (as a start). Schools would not reopen before January 2021.

There was a great deal of criticism about holding the election in a pandemic. Some public health experts recommended against it and chastised us going ahead with it. But there was no telling what would happen with the virus, and the government needed a renewed mandate with the difficult times and the difficult decisions ahead. Though it was pushed by several people on the media, changing the election date was not an option. Once an election is called, it has to be held, as Parliament has been dissolved. In extraordinary circumstances, such as "earthquake, hurricane, flood, fire, outbreak of pestilence or outbreak of infectious disease or other calamity," the constitution provides for one extension of no more than thirty days.

An election was going to be held, in the most extraordinary circumstances imaginable. The upcoming election wasn't the only concern, though it was top of the list. School was set to reopen on September 7, 2020, and a back-to-school grant for students on the PATH and poor relief programmes was announced. That now appeared unlikely.

It was anyone's guess what would happen.

Ring The Bell |

The pending election meant that I had to shift my focus from the MOHW and the COVID-19 response to my constituency. I learned the hard way that being present and visible in the constituency is necessary to retain one's seat. In 2011, I lost my seat by thirteen votes, the main reason being my constituents didn't see enough of me. Being on the ground in West Central St. Catherine wasn't about "COVID stop keep"; it was a pragmatic and necessary step if the JLP were to win the next election and remain in office. My efforts as minister thus far had borne sufficient fruit. There was abundant proof of that. I felt that the management of the pandemic was being well handled by the MOHW, and my not being there around the clock as I had been would not have been detrimental.

Campaigning in a pandemic was different from normal times. No mass meetings, no community events, no rum-shop campaigning. MOHW drew up a campaigning protocol whereby the main activity would be commissioned party workers in groups of no more than five, carrying out door-to-door-type activities. The Electoral Office of Jamaica devised its own election day protocols, involving several steps between arriving at the polling station, casting one's ballot, and dipping one's finger in the ink, interspersed with hand sanitising steps along the way.

Management of the pandemic itself featured prominently in the campaign and was touted as one of the administration's achievements, which it was. Approval ratings for the prime minister were high, the highest of any prime minister in Jamaica's history, the pundits said. My approval ratings were also high. The country had approved of what we had done and how we had done it, even with the mistakes that were made. Despite its earlier efforts at politicizing the pandemic response, the opposition had by then ceded the moral high ground on COVID-19 to the government. Beyond a few people grumbling about it being a wrong time to hold an election and one or two making noise about the rise in case numbers, the opposition's own internal struggles kept them occupied, and they too had to prepare for the election.

By August 21, the situation was so dramatically different it was hard to believe that the election had only been announced ten days earlier. The numbers of positive cases and deaths were unlike anything we had ever seen. Two emergency press briefings were held in five days. The cabinet subcommittee met several times. With stories coming out of Trinidad and Tobago that their spike was attributed to the campaigning surrounding their election, and the basic fact that campaign activities were obviously conducive to spreading the virus, the PM announced new campaign rules: motorcades should not carry general supporters. No buses allowed. Maximum two coaster buses for staff, no more than fifteen in each bus, no hanging out windows, no stopping. The established protocol regarding house-to-house/door-to-door campaigning was amended: campaigners would now not enter anyone's home. They would stand at the gate, wearing masks, having sanitised their hands, and deliver their voters' guides or their paraphernalia.

A new curfew was announced for Kingston and St. Andrew, St. Catherine, and Clarendon. While it was far less restrictive than the curfews in March and April, the restrictions were greeted nonchalantly, unlike the attempt at mass exodus from St. Catherine when they were first put under parish quarantine. The prime minister explained: "The virus only moves with persons, and I have to emphasize this point. The virus cannot move unless we move and so the measures that we are putting in place are designed now to limit movement, to limit unnecessary movement." That the restrictions were less stringent was also a tacit recognition that quarantines were resource intense, and enforcing them detracted from the security forces' other work.

The situation got worse by the day. On August 23, the news broke that the commissioner of police, Major General Antony Anderson, had tested positive for COVID-19. The commissioner was the third high-profile Jamaican to go public. The mayor of St. Mary, Richard

Creary, had shared his positive diagnosis first, and then Chris Dehring, a well-known businessman, went public not long after. Julian Robinson, the PNP general secretary, shared his positive test result. I knew of other politicians who tested positive but felt their re-election would be jeopardized by sharing the news.

Track legend Usain Bolt tested positive the next day. He was to travel for work, and so had taken what he thought was a routine COVID-19 test, which came back positive. It also came to light that the day after he was tested, before he had his result, his girlfriend had thrown him a surprise breakfast birthday party. Videos from the party circulated on social media; few people were wearing masks.

The Bolt situation not only showed that no one was immune to COVID-19, but it also showed how fickle the public is, the vagaries of public opinion, and how social media exacerbates that fecklessness. One day, the timeline was filled with outrage that campaign activities were spreading COVID-19 and how the government was irresponsible to call an election at this time. The next day, the tune changed to how the government is doing its best, and a spike can't be blamed on the campaign, that the surge was due to people's irresponsible behaviour.

In just one month, Jamaica's entire COVID-19 picture had transformed. On August 1, Jamaica recorded, in total, 883 cases of COVID-19 and ten deaths. On August 31, 2,459 cases and twenty-one deaths. In one month, we had more people die than in the entire preceding five months put together, and our number of positive cases was nearly 300 percent higher. We reminded ourselves and the public that what we were experiencing had always been projected. We pointed to the epidemiological graphs that were presented in March and April that showed a sharp spike once an inflection point was reached. We had now reached that inflection point. An inflection point refers to a turning point in the trajectory of the epidemic where the rate of growth of new infections begins to change. (The term *inflection* is used because the change in the rate of growth is often depicted as a bend or curve in a graph showing the number of cases over time). In the case of COVID-19, an inflection point signaled a change in the spread of the virus, and in this case, it meant that the spread had broadened, and more people were getting infected. It just happened later than we had originally expected.

We had the answer to the question that we asked ourselves every day since March 10: "Are we in community spread yet?" Now the question was where to go from here, and who would form the government that would be tasked with answering that question and implementing the answers.

Community Spread |

Friday, September 4, 2020. We were still the government, after a landslide victory. We expected to win, but no one could have predicted the outcome: of the sixty-three seats, we won fifty. We had gone into the election with the house at thirty-three to thirty, and among the seventeen new seats that we won were several upsets of longstanding PNP members of Parliament that no one ever thought could be beaten. The turnout was abysmal, 37 percent, compared to 48 percent in 2016, but the mandate was incontrovertible. The following Monday, September 7, I was sworn back in as Jamaica's minister of health and wellness for a second term, the same day the prime minister was sworn in. The usual large swearing in ceremony was not considered. There was no time to lose. The work had never stopped, and we had a lot of work to do.

Also on September 4, the day after the election, the official declaration was made that we were now in community spread. I made the declaration at a press conference. I also made clear to the Jamaican people that a further surge was expected, given the campaigning and the movement of people on election day.

Community spread is a term with a specific meaning in the context of diseases and epidemics. It means that large numbers of people are testing positive for the virus, and the source or index case cannot be identified. Community spread meant that the source and progress of the virus could no longer be tracked on a case-by-case basis. For several months, we thought that Jamaica had been spared community spread, and we considered this a significant achievement. It was not by luck: there were many cases that could easily have become community spread if we had not identified them early, isolated the patient, quarantined the community, and done intensive contact tracing. One traveler came home to Jamaica with the virus and spread it to each of the five households that he visited on his return. The contact tracers stemmed the exponential spread that would almost certainly have happened had the public health team not gotten to each household. But it was a fantasy that we could stave off community spread indefinitely, no matter what we did.

Post-election we had to deal not only with the changed course that the pandemic had taken but also the political fallout that accompanied it. The opposition began to push a narrative that the government had created an illusion of empathy and transparency, which we abandoned after winning the election. They argued that having won the election, we stopped engaging as we no longer needed to rally public support. Fake news circulated via WhatsApp that Microsoft founder, Bill Gates, bought the election for the JLP so it would have the majority in Parliament and pass a law making it mandatory for people to be vaccinated. None of this was true, but the narrative had to be countered immediately before it grew into public opinion. It would take more than going on radio and denying it. I had to become more visible, among the people, so they would be reassured that we had not given up the fight against COVID-19 because we had won the election. I designed a two-week plan of activities across the entire island as part of that endeavour.

Despite the surge-led spread of the virus, there was sustained pressure to remove restrictions and further reopen the economy. A survey done in June and July found that eight in ten households with children experienced a reduction in income, with households losing an average of 46 percent of their income.[1] If economic needs were not moved up on the priority list, the country would face not only severe economic stress but also its social and psychological consequences.

Even with the surge and the declaration of community transmission, restrictive measures were not reintroduced. We knew those measures would stem the virus's spread, but we were no longer prepared to pay the price that came with them. We were striving for a near-impossible balance: restrictions curb spread but hinder the economy; at the same time, an economy can neither function properly nor recover if the virus is out of control. What then is an acceptable level of infection? There was no formula. Each country weights the different variables according to their own determinations. Countries like New Zealand determined an acceptable level of infection to be zero and imposed some of the strictest measures anywhere, re-instating them when the virus found its way in and began to spread.

Zero was not an option for us. But what was our acceptable level of infection?

By the third week of September, Jamaica counted some seventy deaths and over five thousand cases. We were reporting over a hundred new infections each day, some days over two hundred. These were astronomical numbers to us then. The challenge now: conveying to the Jamaican people that we had not lost control, that the situation we were in was anticipated, and that we were dealing with it, in terms of the public health response, according to best practice.

In a crisis, a government's ability to convince its citizens that a situation is under control is a crucial factor in managing a crisis effectively. A government's credibility and trust among its citizens can help to dispel fear and anxiety, reduce panic and chaos, and increase cooperation and compliance with public health measures. Effective crisis communication and leadership can have a significant impact on public perception and behaviour during a crisis. Transparency, consistency, authenticity, and credibility were all essential qualities and attributes to project and to practice.

We shared with the Jamaican people the truth: our hospitals were equipped to deal with the expected cases needing hospitalization. We had augmented the cadre of contact tracers by several hundred healthcare workers. We were following a testing protocol that, however counterintuitive, was designed to identify the cases where they most likely were. We continued to increase hospital and testing capacity. We were considering participating in a global trial of a Remdesivir, a drug that showed promise as a treatment for COVID-19.[50]

---

[50] The trial was stopped by WHO; they ultimately recommended against its use. Jamaica did not end up participating in the trial as indemnity from the Government of Jamaica was not obtained prior to the trial's end.

The losses were significant. The death toll was not only high; it was hitting home as well. One of the seventy people who died on September 17 was Dr D. K. Duncan. D. K. was a veteran politician, having been member of Parliament in several governments since the 1980s. I was fond of him. I knew him well and considered him a friend. He had been campaigning for the PNP in Central Kingston and Clarendon, where two of his daughters were candidates, as well as across the island for others aiming to hold on to their seats. At eighty, he still loved politics and loved being on the ground. Several candidates and campaign workers contracted COVID during the campaign, but he was compromised by his age.

Another blow was that the reopening of schools that was slated for September was postponed to October. The idea was that when schools would reopen, it would be a blended approach, a mixture of online and in-person interaction. The delay would allow time for the Ministry of Education to source additional tablets and computers to facilitate remote learning. (When the time came, all schools opened remotely, as it wasn't considered safe to open to in-person learning at all.)

No matter how we framed it, regardless of how well we were managing, there was no way to deny or ignore the losses that were incurring. Any notion that we had of getting through the pandemic with minimal cost was displaced by an imperative to staunch the heavy losses and do whatever we could to prevent more. We had work to do.

Being sworn in as health minister for a second term felt like a formality, because the work never stopped, even during the campaign. It's unusual for someone to continue in a portfolio from one administration to the next. But we were not in normal times, and nothing was usual. Though I was continuing in the portfolio, I nevertheless thought about what I wanted to accomplish in this new administration.

COVID-19 was far from over. Although it was the number-1 public health priority, our other public health problems had not disappeared. We simply stopped attending to them. I wanted to re-focus on NCDs, which was still Jamaica's most serious public health problem aside from COVID. Non-communicable diseases compromised people who contracted the COVID-19 virus, making them more likely to fare poorly or even die. But COVID-19 crowded everything else out.

The daily numbers of COVID-19 cases dominated our perspective on how well we were managing and what needed to be done. I had become uncomfortable with defining success by numbers of positive cases, but I acknowledged that I was at least in part responsible for getting us into that trap from early in the pandemic. Numbers were what the general public and the media were using to gauge how well or how poorly we were doing in managing the virus. A truer gauge would have been to look more qualitatively at hospitalizations and deaths and prevention measures. In that regard, we had managed well. Even with the surge, hospitals had not been overwhelmed. We learned that not all positive cases needed to be hospitalized, only the very sick.

Other things were going well. The crisis response had delivered on many fronts. We were strengthening the system's capacity to respond to the pandemic. We employed an additional 121 doctors who were new medical school graduates. We set out to employ additional nurses from the Cuban Brigade. At least 700 of a proposed 1,400 community health aides had been engaged, with the remainder to be onboarded by December. Then 421 additional public health inspectors would be added to the existing cadre. They would be deployed to monitor and supervise the protocols in facilities and work places. Some 1,200 additional patient care assistants would be hired to support the care of patients in facilities.

To address staff burnout, we created a J$37-million staff welfare programme. Among the features of the programme were mandatory rest days, results in forty-eight hours for staff who took COVID-19 tests, special rates at the island's hotels, and family support and counseling, where needed.

And still, the virus raged on. At the end of September, the number of cases had increased to 3,872, the number of deaths to eighty-seven.

Almost 70 percent of cases were from Kingston and St. Andrew and St. Catherine, concentrated in one part of the island, and the idea was to try to keep it that way.

That was not all: the pandemic's other effects were starting to present themselves: the psychological and emotional repercussions of the alteration to normal life and the prolonged dislocation and isolation were showing. It was insult added to injury. It was relentless. And everyone was feeling the strain.

Collateral Damage |

By October, I was tired, the political directorate was tired, the ministry staff was tired, and Jamaica was tired. By this time, we had all expected we'd be well back to normal. But we were far from that. The election should have renewed us with a new, overwhelming mandate, but we were still in the midst of a community spread surge.

Each day, the numbers of positives were in the hundreds. By now, we had just over 7,000 confirmed cases, over half of which were active, and 120 people had died, a fatality rate of 1.7 percent. Our previously lower-than-average death rate had been subverted. Even still, the US and several European countries were experiencing ongoing, unabated surges and far higher death rates.

Jamaica was a mirror image of where we had been in April: major restrictions and few infections then, widespread infections and fewer restrictions now. A split in public opinion had emerged: calls for a new lockdown on one hand, press ahead with opening up on the other. From the government's perspective, a lockdown was out of the question. The strategy was to limit the spread of the virus and manage the risk while maintaining productive activities in a safe way through observing the protocols. Christmas was coming, which would bring opportunities for businesses that had suffered for months. For public health, however, it was not a season to celebrate, but one which was sure to bring a new surge.

Whitfield Town in Kingston and Waterford in St. Catherine, both volatile, depressed, and densely populated communities, experienced outbreaks and were put under a 6:00 pm to 5:00 am curfew for two weeks, from October 6 to 20. But the rest of the country was freed up more and more. The age limit for stay-at-home was lowered from seventy to sixty-five, whereby those sixty-five years and older were required to continue to stay at home but were allowed to leave home once each day for "the necessities of life." In mid-October, the all-island nighttime curfew was relaxed by one hour, from 8:00 pm to 9:00 pm (until 5:00:am the next morning). The Heroes Day holiday long weekend was subject to a 3:00 pm to 8:00 am curfew on Sunday and again 3:00 pm on Monday, the day of the holiday.

The pandemic's other effects were beginning to become clearer. We were seeing psychological and emotional repercussions on the elderly who had been restricted to home since March. They were lonely, some to the point of despondency. Geriatricians reported that their patients were deteriorating far faster than they ought to have. The lack of activity and social interaction for such an extended period had been deleterious for them.

Research findings came in showing that children were psychologically dislocated amidst growing tensions in homes that were now under economic pressure. The COVID slide, the term coined to denote the learning loss that was thought to have occurred when schools closed, was a concern, as it became clear that significant numbers of children had not accessed remote school at all or had not been able to access it properly because of the lack of access to the internet or to an appropriate device. There were suggestions that interpersonal violence was increasing, including domestic abuse and abuse of children.[51]

Second quarter GDP had declined 18.4 percent compared to the second quarter of 2019. Both goods and services had declined (13 percent and 20 percent, respectively). Hotels and restaurants recorded a decline of 86 percent. Even if we had weathered the virus relatively well, we were not spared this collateral damage.

What could we in public health do? The main work of the MOHW at this point was to limit the spread of the virus, including community quarantines where necessary. We were finding it more difficult to enforce community quarantines though. People were less obedient and didn't take the threat seriously. They entered and exited through

---

[51] Caribbean Policy Research Institute, "Socioeconomic Impact of Covid-19 on Jamaican Children," Kingston: CAPRI & UNICEF, 2020.

multiple entry points. A scaled down community quarantine, which was less restrictive, was considered a more practical approach, whereby people would be allowed to go to work, take public transport, carry out their essential activities of daily living such as shopping, visiting the doctor, and carrying on their small businesses.

In a crisis, it is important to be proactive and adapt quickly to new and emerging threats, even while the main crisis is ongoing. We were continually monitoring the situation, looking out for new developments and potential threats. Flexibility was a challenge; whereas a willingness and ability to adapt and respond to new threats is ideal, our capacity issues meant that we were weak in that attribute. We often had the intention, but were without the backing necessary to follow through. We were good on communication, however, and we kept all relevant stakeholders informed and engaged to gather information and build trust. That helped with collaboration. In a crisis, organizations should work together and leverage each other's resources and expertise to respond to new threats, whether in a formal partnership or informal collaborations.

Having realized that there were significant mental health outcomes from the pandemic, a mental health response started in October. We opted to do a volunteer programme, as we didn't have enough community mental health officers, a reflection of the chronic shortage of human and financial resources allocated to mental health. I held virtual meetings with civil society groups across the island, with the objective of getting their support to ameliorate some of the negative psychosocial effects of the pandemic that had been identified. It was a basic concept to get people to visit with and interact with the older population who had been confined to home for so many months and who needed an intervention.

The bureaucracy proved formidable. The volunteers had to have background checks for the ministry to authorize them. For that, we relied on the Ministry of National Security. We ended up with only thirty-five volunteers, and it wasn't until mid-January that they were cleared, and we could begin training. It wasn't the huge effort I had envisioned, nor would it address any meaningful proportion of the people who needed help, but it was a start. In government, the need to cross Ts and dot Is often means that ideas either die, or if they do persist, they manifest in much watered-down versions of what was first put forward. Accountability and procedure are of course important, especially somewhere like Jamaica that has lost so much to corruption, but it was disheartening that the initiative to attempt to address this crucial problem was weakened as it was.

How would we deal with all the collateral effects of the pandemic when it was so difficult to get just one initiative off the ground?

Contagion |

We turned a corner in November 2020, when antigen tests were finally approved for use in Jamaica. They were cheaper, easier to administer, and gave results in half an hour, as opposed to twenty-four to forty-eight hours. They were not as accurate as PCR tests, but they were still useful.

The day-to-day management of COVID-19 was now a routine part of the MOHW's work. The primary consideration in November was the upcoming holiday season in December. The technical team was preparing to propose to the prime minister that the fourteen-day quarantine for incoming travelers remain, that the limit for public gatherings be fifty, and that a curfew continue to be imposed.

Community spread meant that more people were dying, but we continued to avoid some of the horrific scenes that were playing out in other countries. One of the most vulnerable-to-COVID-19 populations across the world was people in long-term care facilities, such as homes for the elderly, and also prisons. In the US and Europe, COVID-19 had been most devastating in such settings. Despite making up just 5.7 percent of all US cases, nursing home and assisted living facilities residents and staff accounted for 39 percent of the deaths.[52] Across the United Kingdom, 28 to 50 percent of all COVID-related deaths occurred in elderly care home residents.[53]

One of the first restrictions enacted was to disallow visits to infirmaries, precisely because the persons there were extremely vulnerable due to their age and health, and also because with so many people in such close proximity, a contagious disease like COVID-19

---

[52] "Covid Cases and Deaths in Nursing Homes Are Getting Worse," CNBC, November 30, 2020, www.cnbc.com/2020/11/30/covid-cases-and-deaths-in-nursing-homes-are-getting-worse-.html.
[53] "COVID-19: Managing the COVID-19 Pandemic in Care Homes," British Geriatrics Society, March 30, 2020, www.bgs.org.uk/resources/covid-19-managing-the-covid-19-pandemic-in-care-homes.

would spread rapidly. Visits to children's homes and prisons had also been paused, for the same reason. That we hadn't had an outbreak in any of these types of facilities was something we congratulated ourselves about, with relief.

Then in October 2020, the Golden Age Home in Kingston, a public infirmary that is the largest care facility for the elderly in Jamaica, with some 450 residents, had eighty-seven positive COVID cases, twenty-two of which were staff members. We felt sure our luck had run out. Of all those who contracted the virus, one resident died, the first person who was diagnosed. This was a remarkable outcome, and a welcome surprise. One month later, there was another cluster in another facility. The Faith Centre, which assisted vulnerable, impaired, and homeless men and was run by the Missionaries of the Poor in downtown Kingston, had a cluster of eighty-eight COVID-19 cases, mostly residents and a few staff. The outbreak was contained. No one got seriously ill, and no one died. Again, we were fortunate. Either of these situations could have had far more tragic outcomes.

The incarcerated population too was a concern, given the inherent susceptibility of people living in such close proximity to each other, with no possibility of social distancing, conditions which were ideal for spreading the virus. In the US, of the approximately 2 million people incarcerated, there were 275,000 infections and 1,700 deaths.[54] In Jamaica, we managed to avoid the virus entering any prisons or jails until October, when a cluster of several dozen people was identified in one of the prisons, mostly staff and some inmates. By early January, of some 3,700 inmates across the island's prisons and remand centres, there had been thirty-nine cases. No one died. Sixty-two correctional services staffers contracted the virus; none of them died either. How we managed to avoid fatalities when these were commonplace elsewhere has not yet been answered.

I was working a dual track: the pandemic and everything else—all the pre-pandemic issues, plus new ones. I resolved to make my time

---

54 "How COVID-19 Has Turned Prisons Into Virus Factories," *Time*, December 28, 2020, https://time.com/5924211/coronavirus-outbreaks-prisons-jails-vaccines/.

at the ministry be about more than COVID. I wanted to re-focus on what was my priority area from the outset of time in this ministry: non-communicable diseases, wellness, lifestyle change, and personal responsibility. I was looking forward to a salts and fats study, an upcoming *Bloomberg* "What's in your food" campaign, and a front-of-packaging food label push.

For COVID-19, I felt my efforts were best spent in raising awareness, morale boosting for healthcare workers, and maintaining public trust by ensuring that the public knew that COVID-19 was still with us and that the government was still actively managing it. That meant being on the road, being present across the island, visiting communities, engaging stakeholders, and motivating frontline workers. There would be life after COVID-19, and the work for that had to go on. The appointment of a state minister, the Honourable Juliet Cuthbert-Flynn, provided welcome support in carrying out the ministry's work. A former Olympian, she was the ideal role model for the health and wellness portfolio.

I was also dealing with my own personal struggles. The year 2020 was one of the most difficult years of my life, maybe the most difficult ever, professionally and politically, because of the pandemic and my position as the face of the response. The upheaval in my family life, though I didn't show it, weighed on me heavily. My sleep was affected, and I often felt burnt out.

We were at a point in the pandemic where we could not see what was coming our way, and it wasn't clear what the way forward was. Nevertheless, we, the government and the ministry, planned as best we could for what we expected in the upcoming holiday season. I tried to put aside my worries and put myself in a more positive state of mind. The results of that effort were mixed. The country's business got done. Me, I was still a work in progress.

Vaccine |

December 8, 2020, brought two welcome developments. It was the day the first COVID-19 vaccine was administered in England, a critical turning point in the pandemic. The creation and distribution of a vaccine was a critical turning point in the COVID-19 pandemic because it provided a tool to combat the virus. Prior to the availability of a vaccine, the primary methods of controlling the spread of the virus were through restrictive non-pharmaceutical measures, such as social distancing, wearing masks, and limiting large gatherings. While these measures were important in slowing the spread of the virus, they also had significant impacts on society and the economy. The vaccine would reduce the severity of the disease in those who contracted it and, it was hoped, would lead to herd immunity, thus extinguish the virus. The availability of a vaccine also brought hope. It gave people a tangible solution for protecting themselves from the virus, and provided leaders and decision-makers with the glimmer of possibility of a road map for returning to normalcy.

Also, on that day Standard and Poor's (S&P) Global Ratings gave Jamaica a B+ rating. In their analysis, S&P stated their expectation that Jamaica would return to fiscal surpluses in the short-term due to the government's demonstrated commitment to prudent fiscal policy management. The report acknowledged the economic fallout from the pandemic, particularly the disruption in tourism and other productive sectors but noted Jamaica's ability to fund the COVID-19 public health, economic, and social response as it did. Jamaica, said S&P, was expected to rebound in 2021 and fully recover in financial year 2022/2023.

The Standard and Poor report was encouraging. An objective entity had essentially measured our performance in all aspects of the pandemic management and found that we had done reasonably well. Few other developing countries had managed their finances as well as we had and hardly any had not borrowed their way through the pandemic. The fact that we had done relatively well in managing the virus, its spread and its damage, was a key factor in this positive forecast. Jamaica's infection numbers and deaths had trended down since October, and while there were several dozen new cases reported each day, the death rate remained low.

Conditions on the ground were looking up. Most businesses across the island had reopened. Traffic was back to pre-COVID normal, or it felt like it was, with rush hour standstills that we hadn't missed. A pilot of face-to-face learning in a handful of public schools had been successful; not a single case of coronavirus occurred, and 109 more schools were slated to reopen in January. A nighttime curfew and gathering limits were still in effect, though these had been relaxed for the Christmas season. Masks were still mandatory, and social distancing was still the order of the day. It was the closest we had been to "normal" since March 10, 2020, and with a vaccine finally created, the expectation was that would continue.

By this time, we had just over eleven thousand COVID-19 cases, mostly locally transmitted. Imported cases were no longer a factor. We had 265 deaths (a 2.4 percent fatality rate), and over 60 percent of the cases were recovered. There was a troubling hotspot, the parish of Westmoreland, where positive cases and deaths had risen sharply since mid-November. A team was dispatched, and detailed mitigation measures planned and started. Stricter social distancing measures were applied, and an expanded curfew was later enacted, which is to say that COVID-19 was still very much with us, but we were coping, and there was no cause for panic or alarm.

The coming holiday season brought many COVID-related considerations. It would be an opportunity for businesses to make some sales before the year was out. Retail, restaurants and bars, and entertainment services had all been among the greatest casualties of the pandemic response. In almost every town, there was a debate about Grand Market. Grand Market is the annual Christmas Eve shopping event held in all major towns across Jamaica, where shoppers have the opportunity to make last minute purchases for the Christmas. People are out and about, and it's usually a festive occasion. The question was: should it be allowed to happen or would it present too great a risk for spread of the virus?

Coming ten months into the pandemic, COVID fatigue was entrenched, and many people intended to celebrate Christmas as they usually would, regardless of the pandemic still going on. We expected tens of thousands of Jamaicans from the diaspora, and when they came, they would not be staying at home quarantining, regardless of the restrictions that they should do so. Our previous surge had happened after a similar holiday period. Another surge was inevitable. It was not a matter of "if" people would flout the restrictions on gatherings, but what we would do when the inevitable surge resulted. The CMO, informed by the data and the modeling, predicted that we would start to see a spike as early as December 15. The US and several European countries were continuing to record high infection and death rates, even higher than the initial stages of March and April. Germany announced a total lockdown for the entire Christmas period.

I launched a new campaign, "Mask up before you talk up," and took it to every parish in the island. I didn't expect that to bring about a turning point, but neither could I do nothing. And so I did what I knew best: go on the road and engage people. Together with public officials such as the mayor and members of Parliament, I walked through the town with the community health aides, carrying placards, and handing out masks and hand sanitiser. There would be a street performer to attract attention and create a buzz. I was visible, connecting with people on the ground and listening. We would never be able to measure the effectiveness of the campaign, but we at least had to try and had to be seen to be doing something. Having covered as many other bases as I possibly could, that was what remained.

Mutation |

It was the Monday before Christmas 2020, and England was again the source of new COVID-19-related challenges. England was where it had all started for Jamaica. Patient One brought COVID-19 with her from England. In the previous forty-eight hours, over a dozen countries had banned travelers from the UK. After a four-week national lockdown that ended at the beginning of December, there was a rapid increase in COVID-19 cases in Southeast England, leading to the discovery of a new variant of the COVID-19 virus—a mutation, as it were. This variant was estimated 70 percent more transmissible than previously circulating variants. The mutated virus caused more serious infections, and it would certainly make the virus's spread less manageable, even with a vaccine.

We remained fairly steady in Jamaica. New cases per day for the previous week ranged from thirty-two to ninety-six, taking us up to just over twelve thousand cases total since the beginning of the pandemic, the majority of them recovered. The number of deaths was the most important indicator. At 286 deaths, we were still on the low end of death rates when compared to other countries.

I met with the technical team at MOHW early that Monday morning. They were working according to the plan to prepare for a holiday surge. From there, I joined the cabinet COVID-19 subcommittee meeting to deliberate on what to do about England. The MOHW technical team recommended a ban. Their presentation summed up what we had learned from all that had happened in the months since the first travel ban at the start of the pandemic and the attempts at controlled re-entry: 1) we did not have the capacity to test at the airports, so a pretest PCR was to be required for residents and non-residents; 2) and we did not have capacity to properly enforce quarantine orders. So it was a ban or nothing at all.

We issued a two-week ban on incoming UK travelers, which had ramifications for the tourist industry, as two thousand visitors who had booked to come were now not going to be able to travel. When the ban was decided, there was already a flight in the air. Passengers on board learned mid-flight that they would have to go into mandatory state quarantine on landing. All 361 passengers were tested. Twenty were positive and placed in state isolation. A few days later, further testing done at CARPHA came back that of the twenty, four carried the mutated strain.

It was an ominous start to the Christmas holiday period. We knew that the relaxation of gathering limits and curfews would mean more mingling of people and higher transmission of the virus. All we could do, however, was wait and hope for the best.

I spent the New Year's holiday with my two sons in Montego Bay. As with most of my personal life since March, they had not gotten the time and attention they needed from me, and I also needed to be with them in that comforting space of family and the people you love. The down time gave me some space to reflect on the year just ended. Certainly 2020 would be a standout year in everyone's lives. No one alive in 2020 would have escaped the pandemic having some effect on their life.

My thoughts were dominated by the job I had done in leading the management of the pandemic. There were some things I felt we could count as wins. We had flattened the curve without going into total lockdown. We held an election and won. We had a surge where for a moment we thought we might have lost control, but the surge was reigned in and the fatality rate remained low. The social and economic dislocation affected Jamaica the most, arguably more so than the illnesses and deaths caused by the virus. The economic fallout, the psycho-emotional impacts, the damage done to children by the closure of in-person school—this wasn't just a conjecture.

Research produced evidence that showed that the worst impact of the pandemic on Jamaica was the economy and on people's mental health. The two were related, as the economic stress directly and indirectly resulted in increased psychological and emotional tension on those who had lost jobs, lost business, or had a pay cut, and on their households and family members.

Our story could have gone differently. Spain, a country with a decades-old universal health system, by mid-December, reported 3,894 cases and 105 deaths per one hundred thousand population (Jamaica had 419 and 10, respectively).[55] The country went on total lockdown for ninety-eight days. People were not allowed to leave their homes, and all but essential services stopped. The spread of the virus was halted, but the economy was devastated. In summer 2020, Spain started reopening, including to tourists, a mainstay of the economy, but within weeks, there was a resurgence, as was occurring throughout Europe. But again, Spain was the worst. Between the high death toll, particularly of elderly people, and the economic devastation, Spain's social fabric was weakened. In assigning blame, divisions were sowed.[56] Jamaica as a country had, so far, held it together.

We could also look to Sweden. One of only a handful of countries that did not go into any form of national lockdown in March and April, Sweden took a herd immunity-type approach, deliberately allowed the virus to go unchecked, and accepted that a lot of people would die, including the elderly. At the outset of the pandemic, many of us looked on at Sweden and wondered if they knew something the rest of us didn't—how could they take such a hands-off approach, while other countries were micromanaging their citizens' and society's every movement? The results after one year were disastrous: Sweden's death rate of over eighty per one hundred thousand people was among Europe's highest and, among its Scandinavian neighbours, ten times as great as Norway and Finland, and over four times Denmark's. By December 21, 2020, Sweden had surpassed the United States and

---

[55] "Coronavirus: Tracking COVID-19 Cases Worldwide," *CNN*, https://edition.cnn.com/interactive/2020/health/coronavirus-maps-and-cases/.

[56] "Spain: More Deaths than Births Last Year for 1st Time," *AP News*, December 16, 2020, https://apnews.com/article/pandemics-coronavirus-pandemic-spain-1ef9868c25c0e2147240d5319dcd0295?utm_campaign=SocialFlow&utm_medium=AP&utm_source=Twitter.

all major European countries in its daily confirmed cases per million.[57] Avoiding stringent lockdown measures did not forestall the economic decline that resulted in other countries.[58]

Though I didn't know it, it was too early to draw any conclusions. The "correct" approach could not be ascertained then, nor for a long time to come. By May 2022, Sweden had one of Europe's lowest COVID-19 death rates, despite shunning most lockdown restrictions, at the time, it was deemed almost to be a rogue state.[59] Even as I write this two years later, there is still no consensus on what was "right," on what counted as success and what counted as failure.

We could, however, see that some of the work that went into responding to COVID-19 would have lasting benefit. The installation of broadband to facilitate remote schooling, the training of teachers in remote learning, the infrastructural improvements in the public health system with regard to new isolation wards and more equipment, and heightened public awareness of the importance of hygiene and infectiousness—these would continue to be valuable after the pandemic and rendered us better prepared for shocks and disasters to come.

There were other positive, less tangible, things that COVID-19 brought about. The pandemic forced everyone to appreciate what they had prior to the pandemic. There was a lot that could be done remotely without the expense and environmental damage of air travel. Those who vacationed overseas re-discovered, or discovered, their own country. All three of these I could speak personally to.

---

[57] "Sweden's COVID Response Was a Disaster. But It's Not the One You're Thinking Of," *Foreign Policy*, December 22, 2020, https://foreignpolicy.com/2020/12/22/sweden-coronavirus-covid-response/.

[58] "Sweden's GDP Falls 8% in Q2, Worse Than Its Nordic Neighbors," *Business Insider*, August 2020, www.businessinsider.com/coronavirus-sweden-gdp-falls-8pc-in-q2-worse-nordic-neighbors-2020-8.

[59] "Did Sweden's COVID Experiment Pay Off?" *The Week*, www.theweek.co.uk/news/science-health/956673/did-sweden-covid-experiment-pay-off.

Because of COVID-19, public health finally got its due. When I was first appointed minister of health in 2016, I had little appreciation for the sector, its importance for national development, and the parlous state of Jamaica's public healthcare system. It was chronically under-resourced and perennially ranked lower than other sectors in terms of priorities for Jamaica's never-enough resources. It took a global pandemic that brought the country and the world to a standstill for the sector to receive long-needed funds for some basic needs and to be considered a priority area for government policy and programming. The fracturing of that old normal, while accompanied by massive societal and economic costs, was a boon to the public health system and was one aspect of the old normal that should never return.

The pandemic also gave the sector and its people a chance to shine. The forecasting capacity and the epidemiology modeling, even where the modeling was off, was critical, as it gave us policy-makers something to work with rather than fumble in the dark. The frontline workers doing the contact tracing and the nurses and doctors in the public system proved themselves. They did the hardest and most tiring work, often at risk to themselves.

Having no idea how much longer the pandemic would go on, I even felt ready to think about the lessons we learned from what we had experienced:

1. **Have a plan**.
    Jamaica didn't have a COVID-19 plan; of course, no one did as it was a new virus. But we did have a detailed pandemic influenza response plan that had been prepared in 2006 and updated in 2007. That plan was based on the principles of rapid implementation of global and national actions, guidance from the WHO and dependence on early disease recognition, high-level political support, and transparent communication—all which we had followed. It was adapted for COVID-19 and gave some structure to what we did, especially in the beginning, before COVID-19 got to Jamaica, and was crucial to our management of the pandemic thereafter. Jamaica

would always have an updated plan going forward, whether for another pandemic or other natural disaster or shock.

2. **Take action early, with an abundance of caution.**
   While the economic and psychological costs were immense, it is almost certain that our early moves to close schools, order people to work from home, to quarantine communities and put people into mandatory quarantine, and to engage in extensive contact tracing slowed the spread of the virus in the first months. The countries that took action early definitely had the advantage in the first stage of the pandemic. Not waiting and seeing, however, comes with knowing that there will be mistakes.

3. **Understand the corollary non-public-health ramifications of any action, and enact mitigating measures at the same time as the public health measures are implemented.**
   Now we knew that economic and social/psychological costs were real and not notional. Going forward, any policy or measure that affects the normal economic and social functioning of society and people must be considered in tandem with those effects.

4. **Stay within the system's existing capacity.**
   Overextending in one area is inevitably going to lead to an imbalance in another area, and it's not sustainable. Again, not a notional concept, but burnout, over-extension, and capacity limitations had damaging effects, especially in a prolonged crisis situation such as was the COVID-19 pandemic. Case in point: testing all travelers as they landed was important at the time to assuage the public that all the sacrifices they had made in staying indoors, and the consequences they had suffered as a result, were not being completely disregarded in favour of reopening the economy, and especially the tourism industry. But it was impractical, scientifically not useful, and led to a backlog in the lab that took weeks to recover from.

Many of those travelers didn't even get their test results while they were on the island.

5. **Emphasize transparency and constant, sustained, coordinated communication, especially repeated breaking down of complex and counter-intuitive situations and policies.**
We understood this from the outset, and we followed through. There has never been such transparency in government business at any other time in our history. Public officials were always available to speak to the media. There were regular press briefings and constant updates to the public. We used social media heavily. Our consistency and openness were laudable, though in retrospect, we could and should have done better on explaining in simple, accessible terms. So much of this new virus and how to manage it was complex, using epidemiological concepts and projections that were often beyond the reach of even medical doctors. Without understanding, however, we risked losing public trust. Testing at the airport was, again, a case in point. In terms of detecting the virus, that testing was not helpful. The nature of the virus was that a person could be carrying it, and it did not show up on a test for several days. So a person with the virus could test negative and go on to develop symptoms and pass the virus along after that negative test. Also, a person could test negative and the next day contract the virus. In terms of a testing methodology, it wasn't useful in showing where the virus was presenting a danger. To establish that, one would have had to test populations that were displaying respiratory illness symptoms, for example, which was what the original testing protocol did.

6. **Collaborate and coordinate.**
For a public sector whose weakness is a tendency to work in silos, the inter-agency collaboration was an achievement, and a necessary one. The field operation was multi-stakeholder and could only be executed properly with support from other

parts of government. The cabinet subcommittee was key to making that happen. The private sector advisory committee was also useful. It was a lot of meetings, and sometimes the meetings went on for hours, but every stakeholder's voice was heard, and input was encouraged.

7. **Preempt staff burnout from the outset by having a predetermined crisis staffing plan.**
   This one would continue to be a challenge in practice, but in theory, I knew it to be true.

I felt satisfied in myself that despite the mistakes we made—and the errors I myself may have committed—there was a great deal to be thankful for. I would come to revisit these in the months and years to come, building on them, tweaking them, adding new ideas, as the crisis persisted.

That contemplative mood and self-congratulatory feeling would be gone less than twenty-four hours later.

Friend |

January 2, 2021, I woke up early to do a five-mile run. As I was tying my laces, I got a message that Tyrone Robinson had died. Tyrone was the chairman of the North East Regional Health Authority (NERHA), the entity that oversaw the public health system in St. Ann, St. Mary, and Portland. He had taken his mother to Miami, contracted the COVID-19 virus, and developed complications. He was only fifty-eight. He had served since 2016, and we all benefited from his passion for public service, particularly in the public health system in the area under his remit. Tyrone was someone I depended on; he gave good counsel, and he was a hands-on chairman who often went out on the frontlines himself to see that things were done. I was floored. I was still absorbing the news when the PS called, with the CMO already on the call.

We weren't forty-eight hours into the new year, and already, it was clear: the pandemic was still a crisis.

After several hours on the phone with the PS and the CMO, we agreed we should do a press conference that same day. There were enough developments that foreshadowed upcoming changes that we wanted to give the public time to brace themselves for what was to come.

First, we needed to ensure the country knew to expect a post-Christmas surge. Several other countries were experiencing some of the worst of the outbreak since the start of the pandemic. In Japan, a surge led to a state of emergency declared in Tokyo and three neighbouring prefectures, amidst a surge in cases and deaths. This was particularly remarkable because of Japan's intense focus on contact tracing, "cluster busting," and widespread mask wearing, among a population that was generally compliant with such requirements and measures.

Second was to address the issue of the new variants. There were three variants of the virus in different parts of the world, all posing a risk to Jamaica. The most likely to reach Jamaica emerged in the UK, what the WHO called the Alpha variant. It was associated with an increased risk of death compared with other variants and had reached several other countries, including the US, by late December. Another variant, dubbed Beta, emerged in South Africa and had since been detected in other countries. A Brazilian variant, Gamma, had also spread beyond Brazil's borders, including to the US. Once any variant was in the US or UK, it was a threat to Jamaica. Ultimately, none of these reached Jamaica in a way that caused a noticeable impact. (It would be a few months later that the Delta variant would reach Jamaica and pose a serious challenge.)

Then other challenges gave us more issues to deal with. The travel ban on the UK was extended for another month. Canada announced that a PCR test was required for all incoming travelers, and there was a possibility that the US might require the same. Jamaica simply did not have the capacity to test outgoing passengers. We had to find a solution. Testing needed to be increased even without that. Budget and finance issues had to be sorted out to ensure that the regions had the resources they would need to continue to deal with all the extra COVID-related demands. Staff burnout and low morale persisted. I wanted to create a welfare programme to address this. I thought some sort of bonus programme for frontline workers should be instituted. I instructed that the ministry ensure that people were taking the leave to which they were entitled. The mental health programme was having difficulty getting launched. And the perennial problem of sustaining an effective communications strategy continued to present itself.

The most important issue of all, and this would largely define the pandemic in 2021, was vaccines. Vaccines were always going to be the world's way out of the pandemic. That it happened in under a year was inconceivable: vaccine development typically takes ten years. The fastest vaccine before COVID-19 was the mumps vaccine, which took four years. The massive investments in and global cooperation for the vaccine's development spoke to the upheaval the pandemic had wrought to the entire world. This was not malaria, affecting only very poor people in a part of the world that was generally outside the mainstream of expensive and intensive medical research. The urgency created by the pandemic across the globe, the serious illness and death rates brought about by the virus, and the devastating effects of non-pharmaceutical measures such as lock-downs led to an acceleration of pre-clinical and clinical trials of potential vaccines.

COVID-19 was a worldwide crisis, and no country, not even the richest, had been spared its devastation.[60]

Vaccines were developed so quickly because there had already been decades of work on a coronavirus vaccine. SARS (severe acute respiratory syndrome, 2002) and MERS (Middle East respiratory syndrome, 2012) were also coronaviruses, and both manifested into epidemics that threatened to become pandemics. Researchers were not starting from scratch when they learned about SARS-CoV-2, the virus that causes COVID-19. Scientists had existing data on the structure, genome and life cycle of this type of virus. It was the previous work on MERS done by scientists at Oxford University that provided the necessary experimental experience and groundwork to develop the very first COVID-19 vaccine.[61] It was an adenovirus vaccine, one which delivers target antigens to induce an immune response. It was the first of several, including other types of vaccines, but it was the first.

A vaccine had been developed, but getting doses to Jamaica was going to be another matter. Jamaica had signed on early for the COVAX facility. COVAX, the abbreviation for COVID-19 Vaccines Global Access, was a WHO-led and endorsed (along with other global organizations) initiative aimed at equitable access to COVID-19 vaccines for developing countries. Where developing countries would not have the scientific and technological resources to develop a

---

[60] "COVID-19 Vaccine Safety," *Yale Medicine*, October 19, 2020, www.yalemedicine. org/news/covid-19-vaccine-safety.

[61] "How Did We Develop a COVID-19 Vaccine So Quickly?" *Medical News Today*, November 13, 2021, www.medicalnewstoday.com/articles/how-did-we-develop-a-covid-19-vaccine-so-quickly#Other-coronaviruses.

vaccine, particularly in the time frame demanded by the urgency of the COVID-19 crisis, the obvious step was for developing countries to pool resources to have a chance at access to the vaccines once they were available.[62] We felt confident in COVAX given that it seemed like a rational, workable arrangement and its endorsement by major multilateral organizations. The original aim of COVAX was to provide vaccines for at least 20 percent of the population of each participating country during 2021.[63] We expected a first delivery of 149,000 to 250,000 doses in February, and by the end of the year, the commitment we had signed on for would see us receiving 450,000 doses.

I shared the news that we would have vaccines by mid-February with the country via an announcement in Parliament. I would later come to regret having made that announcement. Nothing happened the way it was planned, neither the delivery date nor anything that followed thereafter.

The vaccine rollout would entail far more uncertainty than whether or not, or when, a shipment actually arrived. There were other major hurdles. The scale of the logistics of distribution was overwhelming, and that was without taking into account Jamaica's existing poor road and public transport infrastructure. Some of the vaccines required cold storage, an additional challenge given the specialized transportation and warehousing that would be required. There was the question of the manpower to administer the vaccines. Any initiative outside of the regular workload of public health workers—the airport testing, for example—disrupted the entire system as we didn't have enough people.

Most of all, I anticipated we would have a problem getting Jamaicans to take the vaccine. Already COVID-19 had been subject to conspiracy theories, throughout the world and in Jamaica. The nature of the

[62] World Health Organization, "COVAX: Ensuring Global Equitable Access to COVID-19 Vaccines," www.who.int/initiatives/act-accelerator/covax.

[63] "Jamaica Becomes First Country in the Caribbean to Receive COVID-19 Vaccines through COVAX," Pan American Health Organization, www.paho.org/en/news/15-3-2021-jamaica-becomes-first-country-caribbean-receive-covid-19-vaccines-through-covax.

pandemic—lack of certainty about its origins, accusations of "coverups" against the Chinese government, the provisional statements by health experts and authorities that were subsequently updated or even overturned over (mask-wearing, for instance)—gave several openings for conspiracy theorists to ply their trade of spreading misinformation, fueled by social media and instant messaging (WhatsApp in Jamaica).[64] US anti-vaxxers were mobilizing against the COVID-19 vaccine as soon as a month after the pandemic started, and the messages and movement quickly filtered down to us in Jamaica.

The tech innovator turned philanthropist Bill Gates was at the centre of several of the conspiracies in Jamaica; conspiracies which began, it would seem, in the US. The gist of the conspiracy regarding the pandemic was that Gates paid Dr. Anthony Fauci[65] who would, in turn, develop drugs and pass them to drug companies in which Gates had invested. Gates would then guarantee markets in Africa through his control of WHO, which requires those countries to buy the drugs and vaccines. A further objective of Mr. Gates, according to the conspiracy, was to have a premise on which to administer mass vaccinations, and the purpose of that was to insert microchips in people.[66]

I had reason to worry. Despite Jamaica's enviable record of eradication of almost all communicable diseases thanks to vaccinations, and nearly full vaccine coverage of the child population since the early 2000s, we hadn't undertaken widespread adult vaccination since the 1950s (smallpox). The most recent new vaccine campaign, HPV, which began in 2017, had largely been a failure. In 2019, after two years

---

[64] J. Rode et al, "The impact of COVID-19 on knowledge of the electorate." *Nature Human Behaviour*, 2021, www.nature.com/articles/s41562-021-01217-2.
[65] US Director of the National Institute of Allergy and Infectious Diseases and the Chief Medical Advisor to the US President.
[66] "Groups Sow Doubt About COVID Vaccine, One Even Claims It Doesn't Exist," *Loop News* Jamaica, https://jamaica.loopnews.com/content/groups-sow-doubt-about-covid-vaccine-one-even-exists-2.

of vaccinations, Jamaica had a first vaccine coverage rate of only 23 percent,[67] compared to 66 percent in the United States.[68]

In 2020 and 2021, with children out of school because of the pandemic (HPV vaccines were administered to girls through their schools), the first dose coverage was only 3 percent. The rollout of the vaccine on the part of the ministry was flawed, in large part due to the underestimation of the power of social media to transmit the anti-vax sentiment from the US and also from the UK and Ireland. HPV was the first new vaccine since the MMR vaccine had come under anti-vax attack, and in the era of social media. It did not bode well for another new vaccine, particularly given the rampant conspiracy theories already in play.

All of my vaccine worries would prove justified—the logistics, the manpower, and the difficulty in getting Jamaicans to take the vaccine. And even still, there was something else weighing more heavily on me.

---

[67] Global HPV Vaccination Report, "Jamaica," International Papillomavirus Society, https://hpvcentre.net/statistics/reports/JAM.pdf.
[68] US figure is for 2017. Centers for Disease Control and Prevention, "HPV Vaccination Coverage Data and Reports," CDC, www.cdc.gov/hpv/partners/outreach-hcp/hpv-coverage.html.

A Silent Prayer |

I had several things to worry about: the vaccines and all that came with them, a surge which we knew was going to come, daily COVID-19-related crises, the ministry's other non-COVID-19 work, and my work, to which not enough attention was being given. I had lived many lives before I got to the Ministry of Health and Wellness. I was a university lecturer, a policy researcher, a businessman, a cabinet minister in two other sectors, and a member of Parliament for two different poor, rural constituencies. My portfolio responsibility was public health, but my perspective went beyond. All those experiences taught me about what really mattered: people. This was what weighed on me. The toll that the pandemic—the virus and the restrictions—were taking on people was severe.

My concerns for how the ordinary Jamaican was faring were twofold. As minister, I had seen the ravages of COVID-19 firsthand—people barely able to breathe on a ventilator, dying alone, their families grieving. I wasn't only concerned with survival in the physical sense; I was also troubled by the fallout that the pandemic measures had brought, even where I had been the one to advocate for those measures. Outside the hospital, I saw the deprivation and the uncertainty of what tomorrow would bring. For many of Jamaica's poor, survival was about the hustle each day. The pandemic measures had narrowed the scope for that hustle. Business owners, small and medium, were on the brink. The impact on people's mental health was all around me: friends whose children were struggling with online school and being stuck at home and constituents who were depressed and afraid.

For me, the challenge was not only about curbing the virus but also about how we were going to bring about economic recovery. Most other countries were using debt financing to stabilize their economies and relieve their people's COVID-19-induced hardships. Just before the pandemic, Jamaica was emerging from decades of economic stagnation, with one of the highest debt to GDP ratios in the world.

We never wanted to go back there. But might borrowing be a way of mitigating the hardships we were experiencing, and the worse hardships sure to come? Is economic prudence worth social fallout? And if we were to borrow, what would be the best way of utilizing that money? We had done cash transfers, and those helped, but the high informality of Jamaica's economy meant that some of the poorest were not able to access the grants. More hospitals? Investment in employment-generating public works programmes? I didn't have the answers, only several soul-searching questions.

There were no easy answers. There never are.

And then I began getting dizzy spells.

Behind the scenes, there was a lot happening. Tempers were fraying, and the tension was taking a toll. The permanent secretary and I had a falling out, which nearly led to his resignation. It was inevitable that it would come to that, given everything, but it was unpleasant and stressful. I started having episodes where I had a spinning sensation, and I suddenly felt faint. I would have to hold on to something to steady myself. I didn't tell anyone except Dr Carl Bruce, a friend from high school who was a neurosurgeon and now medical chief of staff at the University Hospital. He quietly organized for me to get a full check up with an EKG, a CT scan, and a physical therapy evaluation.

On the day of the tests, I had a scare. The machines had done their bit, and the results were read. I was told to go back to the MRI machine. They had seen something on the scan and wanted a closer look. That was the longest fifteen-minute walk of my life. I was sure I had a brain tumour. A small mass on my brain had in fact been detected. I zoned out as the possibilities of what this might mean flooded my mind. Some minutes later—I don't know how long because time for me had stopped—Carl came back with an old CT scan done several years ago. The same mass was there. Carl concluded it must be a birthmark, nothing to worry about. I closed my eyes and said a silent prayer.

The dizziness, it seemed, was the manifestation of the disruption, uncertainty, and pressure I had been through and continued to go through. I didn't show it, and I never talked about it. Did I even realize it was there? The pandemic and its constant crises, all the other public health issues that needed attention and resources but had been neglected because of COVID-19, my own family problems…it was a lot.

Wallowing and feeling sorry for myself wasn't in my nature though, and it wasn't going to help me, or the country.

I got back to work.

Breaking Point |

By February, we had a goal: 65 percent of the population vaccinated by March 31, 2022. This, we thought, would get us to herd immunity. We would later learn that herd immunity with COVID-19 was not so simple. Herd immunity occurs when a sufficient proportion of the population is immune to a disease, either through vaccination or previous infection, so that the spread of the disease is greatly reduced, and it becomes difficult for the disease to persist in the population. Vaccines that prevent transmission convey "sterilizing immunity"; COVID-19 vaccines did not. While vaccination reduced the chances of COVID-19 being passed to someone else, it did still happen, especially as more virulent strains developed.[69] Though the COVID-19 vaccine did not prevent transmission of the virus, it ought to reduce the amount of virus that is shed by vaccinated individuals, making it less likely for them to spread the virus to others. Regardless, the elderly comprised 70 percent of deaths, so reaching them was a priority. The plan was we would ring-fence the vulnerable (elderly sixty years and over and those with comorbid conditions) and protect them from serious illness with the vaccine. So they would get vaccinated first. Young people were less affected by the virus, and we could afford for them to get the vaccine later.

The rollout was to occur in three phases: phase 1, vulnerable groups; phase 2, those essential to economic activity; and phase 3, the general public. Also, in phase 1 were government officials, healthcare workers, members of the army, the police and the fire service, teachers and school staff, prison system employees, and a few other essential government services.

From the outset, there was a great deal of misunderstanding and anxiety that Jamaica wasn't progressing on getting vaccines. Several

---

[69] CNN Health, "The Myth of COVID-19 Herd Immunity: Why It's Misleading and Dangerous," CNN, https://edition.cnn.com/2022/04/15/health/covid-19-herd-immunity/index.html.

influential stakeholders and stakeholder groups were virtually in a panic, and that anxiety manifested as pressure on the ministry, the prime minister, and on individual cabinet members. The exhortation was to "do something" to get vaccines to Jamaica. In many instances that "something" came with a risk level that we were not willing to tolerate.

I was present to what the vaccine represented and could mean, as were the ministry and the cabinet, but there was a process that had to be followed. We had committed to use only WHO-approved vaccines. We trusted their process and their imprimatur. COVAX too was only going with WHO-approved vaccines. There was pressure to abandon that decision, that it was more important to get a vaccine—any vaccine. We were also being pushed to independently source other vaccines from Cuba and India, and later, Russia. Imagine what it means that there was such desperation that would have led to us using invalidated vaccines. The furthest we were willing to go outside of the mainstream was to explore accessing vaccines outside of COVAX, but only WHO-approved and guided by WHO protocols.

Amidst all the pressure to "do something," people were blind to the reality that the vaccines were simply not available. No matter how much money we had, we couldn't buy the vaccines any sooner than we could actually procure them. It was a rare, but striking example where the lack of resources was not the problem. People were hearing but not listening. When President Biden announced that he was going to get two hundred million more vaccines, he didn't say where he was going to get it from. Many countries would have borrowed or reallocated funds to vaccinate. We would have. But the issue then was access to a safe vaccine. In this way, it was a metaphor for health itself. Sometimes money alone cannot buy what is needed.

And still, my concern was take-up. My inner marketer began to think through what a vaccination campaign might entail: explaining what a vaccine is, the history of vaccines and immunization in human development, herd immunity and the importance of getting a majority of the population getting inoculated. Making clear the benefit of a vaccine to an individual is not readily obvious or relatable, but the impact of this virus is being felt by everyone. We needed to portray a vaccine as the solution, creating hope attached to the vaccine, involving real people from all walks of life to endorse and support. A multidimensional campaign was needed with differentiated messaging targeting specific groups—frontline workers, the vulnerable, the general population. I would be a walking billboard and go out there myself to take my shot and encourage others to do so. I could foresee the first doses being administered—the prime minister and myself, the former prime ministers Patterson and Golding.

The last part of that vision ended up coming true but not in full. When Jamaica finally got vaccines, sometime after we expected, Patterson and Golding were among the first to receive. The PM and I didn't get vaccinated until several weeks after we got the first batch of vaccines. And the first part, the marketing and messaging campaign…that too only partially manifested.

We didn't anticipate how bad the hesitancy would be. As much as I would like to not have regrets, working in advance against hesitancy was one thing I wish I could have done differently. There were anecdotal reports of frontline healthcare workers who were reluctant to take the vaccine. The Western Regional Health Authority did a survey which confirmed the anecdotal reports. And even then, we couldn't have anticipated that doctors and nurses would not take the vaccine in such high numbers. It didn't seem rational: why would people, especially health workers whose profession and training is medicine, not take a vaccine that could save their life? The implications were serious: if frontline people, especially healthcare workers, wouldn't take it, it would send a powerful message and could affect take-up by the rest of the population.

At the other extreme was the desperation to get vaccines by those who did want the vaccine. A CAPRI study would later show that low income and lack of education were correlated with vaccine hesitancy.[70] Those who wanted it were the wealthier Jamaicans, and they were desperate. They used their access to be first in line, whenever they could, creating an outcry that there was unequal distribution of and access to the vaccine.

It was one of the many paradoxes of the pandemic. Some people were going to extreme measures to get a dose and bringing a great deal of pressure to bear to source vaccines, and a whole other set of people were reluctant, and we would be going to extremes to convince them to take the vaccine. None of it was rational, but fear seldom is.

[70] Caribbean Policy Research Institute, "Long Shot: Aiming to Reduce Vaccine Hesitancy," CAPRI, January 2022, https://capricaribbean.org/documents/long-shot-aiming-reduce-vaccine-hesitancy.

Surge |

We were closing in on one year of the pandemic. Something we thought would be for a few weeks, then a few months. One year passed, and there was no indication it would be over any time soon.

Through January 2021, the virus's spread seemed to have leveled off. New infections were recorded every day—about a hundred each day—but the expected, and the dreaded post-Christmas spike had not materialized. Some schools opened face-to-face, and some opened in a hybrid system and were doing a shift or week-on-week-off system (because they didn't have the space to safely have all the students in a classroom at one time). Large hotels were reporting a 60 percent occupancy rate, but several smaller hotels had not reopened at all. Most people were still wearing masks in public; social distancing was still being followed. A degree of normalcy had returned, but there were several sectors that continued to be closed because of the curfews and limitations on gatherings, such as sports and entertainment.

February began with some positive developments. After months of false starts, antigen testing had gotten underway. Private labs could now offer COVID-19 testing, which had been too long in coming and meant a cessation of that set of private sector demands.

But then the numbers began to climb. On February 5, we had the highest number of positives in months, 263. Perhaps it was a blip? We could hope, but we knew that it probably wasn't. Three days later on February 8, there were 328 positives. The virus was not letting up.

The surge was upon us.

We were not alone in the world. Barbados, which managed to open its tourism industry and its schools, including children's sports, and keep its infections and deaths down, went into a two-week nationwide lockdown at the beginning of February, in response to a spike in cases.

Canada, which had been strict about its border closure all along, only allowing in Canadian citizens and permanent residents for most of 2020, found itself in a US-type situation with the spread of the virus getting out of control and several deaths in long-term care (elderly) homes.

Was this a delayed post-Christmas spike? The new more transmissible variants? The alarming numbers reflected several different factors. One was the increase in testing, as private labs had begun providing the service. Another was that people had become complacent, and symptomatic people were not taking precautions at home but were then presenting to health facilities at an advanced stage, having spread the virus to their household and in their communities. The reopening of schools appeared to play a part: though there were no reported outbreaks in schools, the increased mingling of people because of schools being open was thought to have led to an increase in transmission.

The surge gained traction quickly. On February 9, 2021, the prime minister announced in Parliament that the national curfew would be rolled back from 10:00 pm to 8:00 pm. In the broader scheme of the restrictions that we had implemented, this was minor, but it still was a setback for businesses and to the national morale. We hit a new record of confirmed cases: 468 in one day out of a sample of 1,500, a 31 percent positivity rate. We would see some of the highest positivity rates we had ever had since the start of the pandemic.

The outbreaks that we feared were happening all around us. At the women's prison, South Camp Adult Correctional Centre, there was an outbreak, and one woman with comorbid conditions died. At Munro College, a boys' boarding school, twenty-one students and two teachers tested positive for the virus. The Bellevue Hospital (a psychiatric hospital that houses long-stay chronic residents, in a close-proximity-nursing-home-type situation) had over thirty positive cases among its residents, and several staff were also afflicted. We were running out of hospital beds, a critical breaking point that had always loomed, and now it was getting closer. Death rates remained relatively low, but doctors and healthcare workers were strung out.

Their COVID-19 stipend was suspended in January, creating more frustration and withdrawal, and there was an imminent threat that they would lose succor and drop their hands.

Other bad news rolled in that put additional, unwanted pressure on the government. The JLP member of Parliament for Westmoreland Central, George Wright, was accused of beating his girlfriend with a stool after fuzzy video footage was leaked and went viral. That set off a social media frenzy and an internal party debate on how to address what he appeared to have done. I was horrified by what the video footage seemed to show, but I was uncomfortable that within our party, so many people were quick to condemn him without due process. Wright resigned from the party a few weeks after that and became an independent member; he and the woman purportedly in the video announced their plans to marry another few months after that.

Then, just as it seemed things couldn't get worse, there was a data breach in the Jam-COVID border entry screening app. It had been created in record time in the early days of the pandemic to process applications for entry into the country. An American-based tech watchdog, TechCrunch, found that the developer had set the access to the Jam-COVID cloud server to public, and so anyone could access its data without a password. Nearly half a million travelers' immigration documents, passport numbers, and COVID-19 test results could be viewed by anyone. It was embarrassing. There was little I or my team could do. Ministry of Health and Wellness did not own, control or manage the app. It was conceptualized and executed through the Office of the Prime Minister, who had contracted with the Amber Group, a local developer, to create it. The Ministry of Health and Wellness was the target of the vitriol nevertheless, as that was not well understood. When the initial response was deemed unsatisfactory, we were accused of waffling when we had no locus standi to comment. It was resolved, but it made a dent in the effort to build trust.

On top of all this was the J$422-million emergency vaccine communication contract to a marketing company. It was to combat the conspiracy theories and hesitancy that threatened to undermine our vaccination efforts. There was public outrage. The outrage was misplaced and shortsighted, as the majority of the money would pay for advertising space, training, and public education. The company that got the contract would earn J$22 million. While that appeared a large amount to the average citizen, what was to be undertaken was a job that would require a staff with expertise to plan and deploy activities on the ground, and develop content and secure talent for ads, public service announcements, and the like. It would be many man hours, and J$422 million was a good deal for all that we were going to get. But the pushback was weak. I alone defended the contract, but the loudest voices got their way. We were forced to reduce the spend, a decision which many of the same vocal stakeholders who wanted the contract reduced would later come to regret, when it became clear how much of a problem vaccine hesitancy was.

And then another tragedy, another young person lost unnecessarily because of COVID-19. Seventeen-year-old Jalisa McGowan sought medical assistance at the University Hospital of the West Indies for an asthma attack. She was not treated there, and her mother took her to Andrew's, but she died by the time she got there. A three-person review team was appointed to ascertain what happened. The outcome of the investigation found the hospital liable, and they settled with the family. Like Jodian, Jalisa didn't even have COVID-19.

Then the most bizarre incident occurred. Nothing to do with the pandemic, nothing to do with politics. If I hadn't been there myself, I would have found the story unbelievable.

Citizen's Arrest |

Before the pandemic, one of my top priorities as minister of health was the rehabilitation of Cornwall Regional Hospital in Montego Bay. The hospital is large, with four hundred beds, and serves the western end of the island, not just the parish of St. James where it is located. The ten-story building had not been properly maintained since it was built in 1974, and systemic problems had set in. The first four floors of the building were "sick" and had to be evacuated. This had been a problem since at least 2009, but it was only when I became minister in 2016 that the problem began to be addressed. In fact, it was the very first crisis I encountered as minister. I had to decide whether the entire hospital should be shut down.

In 2018, I decided to not shut it down completely. Some parts were closed off, and a rehabilitation initiative began immediately. Several of the hospital's operations had to be moved to outside the main building, to tents, to nurses' and doctors' quarters, and to other off-site health facilities like clinics and smaller hospitals in the area. I visited the site every week so I could personally see the progression. I knew that if the renovation did not have a driver, it would falter.

In December 2019, the projected completion date was the end of 2020. Then COVID happened. And now it was February 2021. There had been cost overruns, faulty work that had to be done over, and the renovation was nowhere near complete.

The project had to be reviewed and revived. I went to Montego Bay to reinject some urgency into it. As I usually do, I organized other meetings on that side of the island around my visit. I met with the chairman of St. Ann's Bay Hospital on the following Friday morning. From there, I went to Trelawney to tour a COVID-19 ward that was being built at Falmouth Hospital. I attended a meeting about the reorganization of the regional health authorities in St. James and then on to Westmoreland to meet with the Western Regional Health Authority chairman.

I stayed the night in Westmoreland at the home of a longtime friend, as I often did when I was in the west. His property was on the beach, and he, myself, and another friend were up late on the beach talking and sharing a drink and chitchat. That type of downtime was like therapy for me, and I got so little of it. Sometime after midnight, in the middle of conversation, my host looked past my shoulder and exclaimed loudly. I spun around to see a tall, strapping young man with dreadlocks approaching us. He spoke English with an accent and said to us that he wanted to make a call. We were shocked but somehow had the presence of mind to apprehend and restrain him in a citizen's arrest. He said he had come from Nicaragua and was having problems. He had come off a boat that was anchored just off the shore. How many more were there? we asked him. Two more, Blu and Luta, he told us. Luta was the captain of the boat. Blu just then came out of the bushes, and we apprehended him too.

They were Nicaraguan drug couriers who had been at sea for three days and had gotten lost. The call they asked for was to their Jamaican contact to ask where to go, to collect "goods" (marijuana), they claimed. They had come to Jamaica on similar business before, they said. This was their livelihood, they told us, how they supported their families. They didn't seem like bad people, just ordinary guys on a hustle. They weren't aggressive or hostile. We made a call to the police and to the army base nearby. Within half an hour, more than fifty soldiers and policemen arrived, everyone struggling to grasp what had really happened. The law enforcement officers were in disbelief that we had apprehended these men without incident. I think they were impressed.

I went to bed at 5:00 am, and when I woke up a few hours later, I wondered if I had dreamt it all. The place was swarmed with police, coast guard cutters, and helicopters overhead searching for Luta. The area was completely surrounded. It was all so improbable—the odds of my being there, of us being up so late, and outside, and then that

I would have anything to do with it. It was like a scene from a movie. They caught Luta later that day. All of them were later deported.

The media found out immediately. With so many people there, it was inevitable. I was bombarded with calls. Social media had a field day. The *Sunday Times* (London) wrote an article about the incident.[71] Things like this you cannot make up, I thought, but immediately, conspiracy theories circulated, including my possible involvement in a narcotics trafficking arrangement. There were accusations that I was out past curfew, that I was at a party, that I was breaching the restrictions. None of it was true. The whole thing was strange, it was normal that people would speculate as they did. I chose to not say anything about it publicly in the hope that the buzz would die down. When asked, I said that it was a police matter, which it was, and there was nothing for me to say.

I still shake my head when I think of that incident.

Next day, I headed back to Kingston—back to reality: the number of new infections, the positivity rate, the reproduction rate. Managing hospitalizations and minimizing deaths had to be considered, along with building new field hospitals, and the psychosocial and economic effects the tightened measures were having. We were under pressure about why we hadn't gotten any vaccines and preoccupied with how we would get Jamaicans to take the vaccine when we got it. And we were about to add regional and international vaccine geopolitics.

---

[71] "Christopher Tufton: Jamaican Health Minister by Day, Crime Fighter by Night," The *Times*, www.thetimes.co.uk/article/christopher-tufton-jamaican-health-minister-by-day-crime-fighter-by-night-62wxjpchk.

Geopolitics |

By the end of February, we were firmly in what can only be called international vaccine politics, or vaccine geopolitics. It was going to get more complicated later, but this was the early days. Countries who were manufacturing vaccines began jockeying for prominence in the vaccine market. It was a commodity that was literally life-saving, which the entire world wanted. This was a once-in-a-lifetime opportunity for vaccine manufacturers.

Countries adopted an "every man for themselves" attitude. Countries would secure vaccines for their own populations first before sharing with other countries. The UK, having been the originator of the AstraZeneca vaccine, announced that they would only begin exporting after their own people had been inoculated. The vaccine was being mass-manufactured in India, and it appeared the UK intended to control access to those doses too. I knew from credible sources that there were problems in Canada, as the US had diverted vaccines that Canada ordered to their own population. The Canadian government was threatening to sue the US.

In our region, Barbados received donations of a few thousand vaccines from India, China, and Russia, including some which had not been WHO-approved when they first landed in Bridgetown. Prime Minister Mia Mottley positioned herself as the person who brought vaccines to the region and offered other Caribbean countries who had not yet gotten any vaccines some of what her country received. She offered Jamaica one thousand doses. We did not accept as we were due to receive a shipment soon. And in any case, one thousand doses wouldn't go very far in Jamaica.

But it stung, and it raised the anxiety of the Jamaicans who had become obsessed with getting the vaccine. Here were much smaller islands—Barbados, St. Lucia, and Grenada—already vaccinating its citizens. People said they felt embarrassed. The pressure increased:

"Why are they vaccinating and we aren't?" "Jamaica is lagging in the Caribbean!" "Why don't we have our act together when others do?"

We repeated our position that we would follow WHO guidelines, that the vaccines the other islands were using were not WHO-approved. It was a painfully ironic situation that we were caught in: we were exercising caution and ensuring that we had safe vaccines that people would trust. That caution was being seen as us having "dropped the ball." That was the expression the detractors repeated: Jamaica had dropped the ball on vaccines.

People were agitated. I was frustrated.

The frustration was about to increase.

I wanted to explain to all of Jamaica what was happening with vaccines. I wrote a piece that listed the reasons we had not yet gotten vaccines, and I answered some frequently asked questions. It was an opportunity to set the record straight and take control of the narrative. On the last day of February, the Sunday *Gleaner* published my op-ed article on vaccines:

Setting Records Straight on the COVID-19 Vaccine[72]

That a COVID-19 vaccine is the light at the end of the pandemic's tunnel is a truth universally acknowledged from the outset of the COVID-19 pandemic. Wealthy countries' governments supported and subsidised the accelerated development of a vaccine, and less wealthy countries, like Jamaica, put their lot in with the COVAX consortium, by contributing an affordable amount of money to a common fund that would also be put towards vaccine development, and would guarantee some vaccines once it was approved.

---

[72] "Christopher Tufton: Setting the Records Straight on the COVID-19 Vaccine," Jamaica *Gleaner*, https://jamaica-gleaner.com/article/commentary/20210228/christopher-tufton-setting-records-straight-covid-19-vaccine.

Jamaica's participation in COVAX was not only meant to secure access to vaccines, but to secure access to World Health Organization (WHO)-approved vaccines. From the outset, Jamaica has followed world standards in the management of the pandemic: our testing protocol was based on the WHO recommendations, our discharge criteria were informed by WHO research and analysis, and our treatment protocols have followed the WHO's evidence-informed guidelines. We trust the WHO's expert panels, including the Strategic Advisory Group of Experts on Immunization.

While many people accept that a vaccine is essential to stopping the spread of COVID-19, not everyone intends to take it. In Jamaica, low take-up of the COVID-19 vaccine would forestall us getting to herd immunity, and the virus would continue to spread, causing illness, hospitalisation, and death. We have reason to be concerned about low take-up as the anti-vaxxer movement has grown and strengthened over the past few years. We have seen this manifest in Jamaica already with the HPV vaccine, where the take-up was less than 40 per cent, despite the vaccine being promoted by all the medical groups in the country, provided free of charge, and protecting girls from a deadly cancer.

Further, the conspiracy theories surrounding COVID-19 include those about the vaccine, and many Jamaicans, including front-line healthcare workers, have implicitly or explicitly stated that they will not be taking it.

Not every vaccine is certain to work. Australia had reserved 51 million doses of a home-grown vaccine that failed in clinical trials. Sanofi and GlaxoSmithKline Plc had to delay their clinical trials after setbacks. Merck shut down its vaccine programme three weeks ago after lackluster early results.

Given these pre-existing factors, Jamaica took the decision that it would only administer vaccines that had passed the strictest international standards. The risk of bringing in a vaccine about which there could be any doubt is too great. Besides compromising this COVID-19 vaccine effort, it could damage Jamaica's vaccine programme for generations to come.

Why have other countries received the vaccine before JAMAICA?

There are three reasons. First, rich countries have accumulated extensive supply deals. The United States struck unilateral deals for all of its 1.2 billion dose supply, four times more doses than its population. Wealth has moved some countries to the front of the line. Other countries may have to wait until 2022 or later before supplies are widely available. Some of these countries have higher rates of COVID-19 mortality and have signaled that they intend to eventually share these enormous supplies.

Second, this hoarding by rich countries has slowed the COVAX facility's obtaining what had been allocated to them. Third, other countries are not following as stringent standards as we are in Jamaica, and are administering vaccines that are not WHO-approved, or yet to be WHO-approved.

Barbados, Dominica and the Dominican Republic received supplies of the Oxford-AstraZeneca produced by the Serum Institute of India through a donation from India, amounting to 100,000, 70,000 and 30,000, respectively. India should be commended for this donation to our Caribbean neighbours. Through this supply, Barbados has vaccinated about 14,000 persons. Some countries, including Guyana and Trinidad and Tobago, have received a small supply as gifts from Barbados. Dominica also made donations to some of the smaller Caribbean islands, including St Lucia, Antigua and Barbuda, St Vincent and the Grenadines, St Kitts and Nevis, and Grenada. St Vincent and the Grenadines also received 20 doses of the Russian Sputnik vaccine, an intermediary dose. This vaccine has not been approved for emergency use by the WHO. Britain and the Netherlands have also supplied their overseas territories in the Caribbean with approved vaccines, including Pfizer and Oxford AstraZeneca.

All Caribbean countries have signed up under COVAX and like Jamaica are seeking to secure supplies from other countries, including China, India, Cuba and Russia through bilateral negotiations.

Jamaica should receive its first supply of vaccines through COVAX by the end of February. A budget of J$5 billion was approved that will allow us to purchase more than three million vaccines. In sum, we will receive vaccines from five sources: COVAX (AstraZeneca, SK), AMSP (AstraZeneca & Johnson and Johnson), India (SI), Moderna (Moderna), and the Jamaican private sector (AstraZeneca, SI).

Vaccine challenges not unique to Jamaica

What we are witnessing across the world is 'vaccine nationalism' instead of vaccine equity. Some countries have cornered the supply so much that they can offer up to four doses per person, while many developing countries are yet to receive a single dose of vaccines. Even where supplies had been secured, several Latin American, Caribbean, and African states do not have enough for the majority of the population. Statistics from Duke Global Health Innovation Centre show that total worldwide confirmed purchases are concentrated in high income (4.6 billion doses) and middle-income countries (1.2 billion doses). This is also true for vaccine administration so far.

What GOJ is doing in the interim

Preparations are being made to ensure that there are no major challenges when the vaccines arrive in Jamaica. Storage and other facilities have been put in place and nurses, who will carry out the inoculation, have been trained.

Despite the human-resource challenges that we face, while we await the vaccines, we are meeting the current challenge by recruiting new staff across the different regions. At the same time, we continue to lose our nurses to richer countries, such as the United Kingdom which has deployed a fast-track (within three weeks) visa recruitment strategy to attract them during the COVID pandemic. Our own recruitment strategy to fill current gaps is therefore extremely important.

The Ministry is also accelerating the expansion of numbers of COVID-19 hospital beds across the island. Field hospitals are being built at Falmouth Public General Hospital in Trelawny, at St Joseph's Hospital & Medical Centre in Kingston, and at the Mandeville Regional Hospital in Manchester. The 40-bed field hospital that was originally sited at the National Chest Hospital will be moved to Spanish Town.

We are expanding our staff capacity to respond to increases in hospitalisations and the resulting pressure on the healthcare system. We continue to focus on testing. Private labs across the island are now certified to conduct COVID-19 tests, and systematic testing throughout the island's hospitals and health centres is ongoing. A nationwide communication campaign is in the works. This is necessary to ensure that every Jamaican understands and appreciates the nature and severity of the problem, the importance and safety of the vaccine, the solutions to the challenges we face, and their role in the process. The campaign will help to bridge the gap between policy and implementation and between the Government's action and that of our citizens.

The Government cannot meet the challenges alone. Citizens must play their part, too. Without compliance with DRMA regulations, we risk undermining the efforts of the Government. These regulations will not be effective if people do not comply.

We must continue, as a country, to make every effort to reduce the spread of COVID-19 and bring the pandemic under control. The Government continues to develop and implement the necessary policies and strategies, but the public must play its part by observing protocols and regulations, wearing a mask, sanitising regularly, avoiding crowds and gatherings, and staying six feet apart from other people. The only way out of this pandemic is for all of the country to be a part of the effort.

Let That Sink In (March 2021) |

The debate continued about how to fix the economy and address the social issues that the pandemic had worsened. The economic model we had been pursuing for the previous six years served us well. We reduced our debt to GDP, which was a significant step that led to the country finally having realistic potential to realize economic growth. That model included practicing fiscal restraint, and the general consensus was to continue to follow that model despite the extraordinary situation of the pandemic.

I felt that there was an argument to be made that the solution in this one-in-a-hundred-years situation was not to fully subscribe to the low-debt-to-GDP model that was used pre-pandemic, but to do what was necessary to keep the population safe and keep them feeling safe. The three largest sectors in Jamaican economy were down—tourism, BPO (business process outsourcing), and the informal economy. Only remittances were flourishing. In that environment, should fiscal discipline be the absolute priority? Was austerity a suitable approach in this extraordinary moment? At times I felt the need to push back on the consensus.

There was also a view that the measures to restrict movement to bring the infection rate down should be loosened, even though we were in the midst of a surge. That the economic cost was too high and there was no evidence that shutdowns worked were the arguments. I often offered a counter to this, sometimes with success, other times not so much. Lockdowns and movement restrictions did work to reduce the spread of the virus; that was indisputable. There were economic and social costs to that, I argued, but those were less than the illness and dying that would result from the continued spread of the virus. Not everyone agreed.

There became a circular argument that went something like this:

A: "We don't have the money to respond to public health and people's needs. We must open up the economy."

B: "Funding for public health interventions should not be dependent on curfews."

A: "The suffering wrought by the virus is less bad than the social and economic fallout caused by movement restrictions."

B: "The continued spread of the virus will result in widespread death and morbidity, which will not only cost us more in public health spending, but will bring about social unrest."

A: "We will have social unrest from people's pent up frustration at being forced to stay home, and being unable to hustle to survive."

It went around and around.

In my head, there was another set of thoughts circling:

- What was fueling the surge?

- We had sent samples to CARPHA to see if the variant was present.

- How do we resolve the concern around getting vaccines?

- Continue with the push to get as many vaccines into the island as soon as possible.

- India had committed to a donation, and we were due an allocation from COVAX.

- How to address concerns and issues that the social and economic costs of restrictions are worth it?

- Constant reassurance that the measures are worth the fallout.

- How do we deal with the hospitals getting filled to capacity with COVID-19 patients?

- Do we need more beds? We were about to add 133 across the island, that should give some breathing room.

- How to treat with the looming vaccine hesitancy?

- There has to be a marketing campaign.

Then I got out of my head and got on with it.

On March 10, 2021, a year to the day that the first COVID-19 case was confirmed in Jamaica, the first COVID-19 vaccines were administered across the island. Two days before, Monday, March 8, Jamaica received its shipment. The government of India donated fifty thousand doses of the AstraZeneca vaccines. They were received at the airport as if they were a visiting head of state. The prime minister, the minister of foreign affairs and foreign trade and the Indian high commissioner, Rungsung Masakui, were there to greet the plane on the tarmac. This is how significant it was.

Marcia Thomas-Yettman, a public health nurse who confessed to being "afraid of injections," was the first to receive the COVID-19 vaccine. She received the vaccine at the Good Samaritan Inn, a faith-based centre for the homeless in downtown Kingston. Frontline healthcare workers across the country received first doses. The former prime ministers PJ Patterson and Bruce Golding were among the first to be vaccinated. Their age put them in the "vulnerable population" category, though both men were quite healthy and fit. Them being among the first was a deliberate attempt to show high-profile people taking the vaccine, in the midst of the growing anti-vaccine sentiment.

The virus was still running loose. The day before the vaccines arrived, our new case numbers were 723, taking us to a 36 percent positivity rate—a record high. I announced the numbers myself and made an impassioned post on social media imploring people to follow the protocols.

"Let that sink in," I said.

> ....
>
> Let it sink in that the positivity rate means that our hospitals are going to come under pressure, significant pressure. Let it sink in that our public health workers, our nurses, our doctors are going to find it difficult to cope with those who come in and need medical care. Let it sink in that it means longer waits, it means persons having to suffer for longer periods before they can get a bed, and generally speaking, a health system that is going to experience significant stress and fatigue. I accept that the Government has a responsibility, but let us be clear that a lot of the spread that is taking place in this country is because too many of us are ignoring the need for personal responsibility.
>
> ....

Immediately, there was a backlash. People took issue with the refrain, "Let that sink in." I was accused of gaslighting. But I was not sorry. I had no intention to offend anyone, but it was time for Jamaican people to hear the truth, that blame for the out-of-control spread of the virus had to be shared by the people themselves. The government, the Ministry of Health and Wellness, could and should not shoulder the responsibility for the shocking numbers. Personal responsibility, a mantra I had been preaching since I first became minister, had to be seen as key to stopping the virus's spread.

The following day, new COVID-19 case numbers were at 878—a new high. I could only hope that something would sink in.

Priorities |

The initial plan was for the prime minister and me to be vaccinated that first day. For the symbolic value with regard to the message being sent to the public and for practical reasons, because we were both out on the road and exposed to the virus every day. Any member of Parliament (MP), to do their job, has to be on the road with people. But vaccines were scarce. The question of who should receive them quickly became politicized.

The priority group, at first, was public sector workers, MPs included, about four hundred people in total. Several other categories of frontline workers were added, taking it up to several thousand. The prospect of so many getting vaccinated ahead of vulnerable groups became a problem. The question was asked by a popular media personality, Dionne Jackson-Miller: why was the prime minister going to be first in line to get a vaccine? Social media picked it up. An uproar ensued. There was internal consideration, especially about the optics of us (MPs) going first. The prime minister decided we would go after the priority groups and so a new listing of who was to be vaccinated was issued:

> After the vulnerable groups of elderly persons...then, the Jamaica Fire Brigade, Department of Correctional Services, Jamaica Customs Agency and Passport, Immigration and Citizenship Agency and workers in educational institutions at the Early Childhood, Primary, and Secondary Levels. Public sector workers who interface directly with the public in the course of service delivery, to include cashiers, customer service agents, transport inspectors, JUTC bus drivers and conductors, case officers, and other such personnel. Government officials, to include Members of Parliament, the Judiciary, Parish Councillors, senior civil servants, and senior technical officers will gain access to vaccines after the priority groups listed above.

I confess, I was disappointed. I had been looking forward to getting vaccinated, given my daily exposure to large numbers of people, including healthcare workers. It was a miracle I hadn't yet contracted the virus, even though I had been careful with mask-wearing and hand-sanitising, given how I had been so exposed. My friends and family were upset and badgered me to "do something." It's always I should "do something." They had been worried about me all along, and now here was a chance to lower my risk, and I wasn't able to avail myself of it. The chatter around the issue was becoming a distraction.

A week after the Indian gift of vaccines arrived in Jamaica, on March 15, 2021, we received 14,400 doses of COVID-19 vaccines through the COVAX Facility, one month late. They had not expected the vaccine nationalism and hoarding. That 14,400 we received was going to expire in one month, but we accepted it and used it up well before the expiry date.

Getting those vaccines represented a marked shift in the discourse around the pandemic and around the ministry's work. The task was not only about prevention, bed space, and treatment. The pressure to get the vaccines into Jamaica now shifted to getting the vaccines into people. The vaccination campaign would be the largest logistics exercise and mobilization effort ever carried out in Jamaica. Whether we would meet the challenge, whether we had the capacity to do this and do it properly, remained to be seen.

On March 19, I received my first dose of the vaccine at the Spanish Town Hospital, on my way to my constituency. With the new batch of vaccines on hand, it was decided that members of Parliament would in fact get vaccinated as a priority group. Getting vaccinated was a relief. I was now more protected; if I contracted the virus, my chances of getting very ill were lowered considerably. My colleagues on the frontlines were also protected. The distracting chatter about whether and when I should be allowed to take it was silenced.

It was a pinprick of light in an otherwise difficult period. The surge continued. We would later call it the "second wave," but we didn't know then that there would be a third wave. We had a 42 percent positivity rate in mid-March. More younger people were dying than before. Contact tracing was hardly relevant with this scale of spread. Hospitalizations and deaths were worrying, not only for the loss of life and the distress to those who had the virus, but also for the first time, I was genuinely concerned that people would die because of the system's lack of capacity to respond and treat them.

It seemed I was to blame for it all. I felt like the public held me responsible, and I knew that many influential people did.

Was I responsible? Was this my fault? Was this the outcome of my decisions?

Just as the vaccination question was settled, an oxygen problem arose. Hospital oxygen was a problem. For someone badly ill with COVID-19, oxygen is essential to keep them alive. It is also used routinely in hospitals during surgery and in treating patients. Over the weekend of March 12 to 14, 2021, we had to announce a suspension of elective surgeries and a halt on all but emergency admissions to conserve oxygen for use in critical cases. The island's sole manufacturer and supplier of medical oxygen, IGL, a Trinidadian company, had difficulties delivering and storing the oxygen, especially where hospitals didn't have onsite storage facilities and internal transmission pipes. Those hospitals took the oxygen in cylinders, and those too were in short supply. More cylinders were to be imported.

It was a fraught three days. Cylinders of oxygen were frantically moved from one hospital to another. This was the closest we had come to the system collapsing. I was actually scared but endeavoured to radiate calm as I fielded panicked calls. I barely slept. Finally, the shipment arrived. It was as happy an occasion as when the first batch of vaccines landed. Whether anyone died because of that shortage was not conclusively determined, but that was something that should not have happened.

Other challenges loomed. As hospitals filled and more beds had to be added, doctors began threatening to resign over the working conditions. A drug that had seemed to offer treatment for COVID-19, Remdesivir, was found to be ineffective in shortening the duration of the illness and was discontinued in Jamaica. Alternative remedies and treatments proliferated.

Ivermectin became an issue of contention. Doctors and the public had been advocating for its use and for the ministry to grant a permit to import it since March. Merck, the manufacturer, put out a statement that the data did not show Ivermectin is effective to treat COVID-19. The ministry's own research found that there was not enough information to recommend for or against the drug for use in COVID-19 treatment. While the MOHW would not bring it in, people could use it if they wanted to. The ministry not bringing in the drug, however, meant a substantial price difference than if they were. A lobby formed around that.

Towards the end of March, infection rates began going down, but slowly. The reproductive rate went from 1.1 to 1.3, but the absolute numbers weren't showing the big decreases that people wanted to see after so much sacrifice with curfews and lockdowns. The surge's longer-than-anticipated perpetuation and the accompanying restrictions led to frustration among everyone—decision makers, healthcare service providers, and citizens. People were fatigued with life in abeyance. Doctors and nurses were burnt out with the heavy workload, and decision-makers were beleaguered by the uncertainty and volatility.

The prolonged surge created an impression that the movement restrictions were ineffective. That was not the case. At the outset of the pandemic, our epidemiology team projected Jamaica would get to a positivity rate of 30 percent, with 450 people ill enough to be on ventilators. It took a year to happen, but it was now playing out almost exactly as had been predicted. It also meant that those early movement restrictions and interventions had worked, that we had managed to disrupt and flatten the curve, or we would have experienced a surge much earlier when the hospital system was still lacking the necessary capacity.

There was one hopeful development, the creation of an electronic payment mechanism connecting customers with food vendors, including small and informal business operators such as pan chicken men, many of whom it was assumed were unbanked and not online. The E-commerce National Delivery Solution (ENDS) was especially useful and important as it allowed vendors to operate during curfew hours, and was a partial remedy to the loss of business in that sector that the movement restrictions had wrought.

The scenario occurred to me that with the vaccines, there would be an expectation that the pandemic's end was near, people might abandon precautions, and the virus would continue to spread. It was not yet time to behave as if things were back to normal.

I realized I was overthinking.

Or was I?

Were we losing this battle?

Was it lost before we entered the fray?

Was I losing my mind?

That is how it felt.

Approved |

We had received vaccines, but were far short of what we needed. Sixty-four thousand people had received a first dose of AstraZeneca. That was a tiny percentage of our target. We still needed to get more vaccines into the country as soon as possible.

The debate shifted to approved versus unapproved vaccines. The ministry and the prime minister were solidly pro-WHO-approved, as was I. (Cliff Hughes would later say that the ministry and I "slavishly" followed WHO guidelines.) The credibility of our immunization programme had been built on WHO guidelines and vaccine approvals. To endorse and administer a vaccine that had not gone through the WHO approval process would be unusual for us. Particularly given the widespread skepticism about the COVID-19 vaccine, we thought it would be a mistake to introduce any vaccine that wasn't WHO-approved, and that administering unapproved vaccines would give fodder to the anti-vaxxers. If our credibility was brought into question any at all, it would be difficult to champion the COVID-19 response.

The counter-argument was that we were behind in the line, and Jamaica was late compared to other Caribbean countries. Strictly speaking, this was not true. We were the first to receive from COVAX; all the other Caribbean countries had been gifted their vaccines. Those gifts had the additional effect of creating the perception that vaccines were available when they weren't. Further, many of those Caribbean countries were administering non-WHO approved vaccines. In any case, it wasn't a race. We would all get vaccines; whether one island got a week before another was inconsequential in the big picture. The "approved only" faction held firm.

We—in Jamaica and surely in several countries around the world— were operating on the premise that the world would come together and recognize the importance of vaccines being distributed equitably and that the world would be better off the more people vaccinated.

But what happened was the panic around the virus created a much more nuanced perspective characterized by "How do I take care of my own?" as if taking care of one's own would equate to things returning to normal. The world was too interconnected for that. What transpired instead was inequitable distribution and hoarding. The first sign of that was the delay in COVAX, when we were told we would get an amount by a certain date, and we got less than that amount and one month late.

The debate was complicated by a misunderstanding of what was happening in the vaccine market at the global level. The manufacturing companies and brands recognized that in months to come, the alignment of supply and demand was going to change. At that time, 9 billion doses were on order and 2 billion in circulation. Demand vastly exceeded supply, but in a few months, that would flip. Vaccines were commercial goods, not just a public health or humanitarian issue. Drug companies appeared to be exploiting the panic and desperation by asking for high prices and commitments to large quantities. They were approaching vaccine sales and distribution from a business modeling perspective, given that in time, the prices would fall so they were trying to lock countries into high prices. I found it distasteful, and I thought it was dangerous. My idealistic view was that there are times when the greater good of the world's population ought to take precedence over drug companies' financial return.

My idealism counted for naught. These were machinations that were well beyond anything under or even near our control, and we had no choice but to be patient while aggressively pursuing several leads, all at the same time. We were grateful to India for the 50,000 doses, happy for the 14,000 doses from COVAX, and we were due another several thousand doses from COVAX in the first week of April. The Africa Medical Supplies Platform (a not-for-profit COVID-19 -specific initiative launched by the African Union), another arrangement we had signed on to, was to send us a token amount of Johnson & Johnson vaccines ahead of substantially larger shipments some months later.

I stopped worrying we wouldn't get vaccines. I figured that vaccines would be scarce for the next couple of months because of limited approvals and less-than-optimal manufacturing capacity. In two to three months, however, I was certain there would be more availability and prices would come down. But while we were forced to bide our time, I did not like the pressure. It was wasted energy.

The goal of 65 percent of the population vaccinated in one year was something I thought about a lot though. I felt we were being overly ambitious. That was what was needed for herd immunity, or so we thought at the time. If we could just get the vulnerable ones vaccinated, I thought. Younger people who didn't take the vaccine would likely get the virus and develop a natural immunity. So we might get to herd immunity anyway.

I allowed myself to imagine…if that happened, and we didn't have another surge, we could be back to pre-COVID-19 normal by 2022.

On that, I was mostly right.

Blitz |

Vaccines came from unexpected places, for unanticipated reasons, and under extraordinary conditions. South Africa halted its rollout of the Oxford-AstraZeneca vaccine in mid-February 2021. It was shown to not confer adequate protection against the new COVID-19 variant there. One and half million doses had been procured for healthcare workers but were now useless to them. The vaccines were perfectly good and could be administered elsewhere, wherever that mutation was not virulent. They sold most to other African countries. By the end of March, however, they still had seventy-five thousand doses. They were going to expire soon, and they didn't want to dispose of them when so many countries were in need. The head of the African Medical Supplies Platform reached out to Jamaica and offered us the vaccines for free.

The chairman of the National Health Fund (NHF), Howard Mitchell, had been tasked with sourcing vaccines for Jamaica. He attended cabinet with the CMO on March 29, a Monday, with a proposal to accept the vaccines. We had been given expert opinion that based on an extrapolation of the data, the vaccines could be used past their expiry date. We submitted that to the WHO, assuming they would confirm. Cabinet agreed, and we accepted the donation. The seventy-five thousand doses of AstraZeneca were dispatched from South Africa on a chartered DHL flight, at a huge cost, which we bore, some US$200,000. This was how much we wanted those vaccines.

Of course. there was the question: how were we going to get seventy-five thousand people to take the vaccine in such a short period of time? We ourselves didn't think it possible and figured that we might use half. We offered Trinidad some, but they also had vaccines that were about to expire. We negotiated with the one of the cruise lines to lend them twenty thousand doses that they could use then, and they could repay us when they got their allocation, but that fell through as they said they preferred Pfizer.

My idea was to take an election campaign approach. Cabinet approved us to give $500,000 to each MP and $250,000 to each councillor to get their people out, as they would on election day. Not only was that a proven way of mobilizing people, but it was also more equitable. This approach meant that people who would have had limited access to transportation, poorer people, people in rural communities, could get vaccinated. Up to that point, appointments had to be made online, which automatically excluded anyone who didn't have online access or a device. Mainly people who had cars or who could go in taxis had gotten vaccinated up to that point.

Desmond McKenzie, the minister of local government and a veteran MP, was in charge of the political mobilization. Juliet Cuthbert-Flynn, the state minister of health and an MP, was assigned to take charge of one set of parishes, and others were assigned to Senator Natalie Campbell-Rodriguez. Those three, together with members from the regional health authority boards, comprised the committee that organized the disbursement of the money through the parish councils and oversaw the mobilization effort.

When the vaccines landed in Jamaica on April 7, a Wednesday, the WHO advised that they would not endorse an extension of the April 14 expiry date. We had not expected this. It meant we had less than one week, a far shorter window in which to administer the vaccines. Up to this point, we had insisted we followed WHO guidelines. We couldn't now disregard them because they didn't suit us. What had we gotten ourselves into?

There we were, on that Wednesday, with seventy-five thousand vaccines that had to be used by the end of the day the following Tuesday. Five days. We determined we would go all out to administer as many of them as we could before they had to be dumped.

Thus was born the first vaccination blitz.

Changes were made to the original plans for this rollout. Announcements were made that tourism workers and teachers were now in the priority groups eligible to receive vaccinations. The instruction was given to the public health teams at the vaccination sites that despite priority groups having been named, anyone who showed up was to get jabbed, regardless of age or category. One did not need an online appointment: people were to be given the vaccine once they presented themselves.

The blitz was to start on Saturday, April 10, 2021, but the ministry's online appointment system accidentally took appointments for Friday, the day before, and eight hundred people had signed up. Cancellation messages were about to be sent out. I said, "Wait!" Up to the broadcast of COVID-19 Conversations that Thursday evening, it was going to be cancelled. I insisted they go ahead on the Friday. Doctors and nurses had to be pulled from health centres, and the National Arena had to be readied. The blitz got off to a rocky start as we weren't fully prepared. But we couldn't afford to cancel, make people feel disheartened, and risk losing their willingness to come back. We inoculated more than the eight hundred that Friday.

On Saturday morning, I set out, heading west. Juliet, Natalie and the CMO made their way to different locations across the island. I planned to make my way to Westmoreland, stopping all along the way, circle back around the eastern end of the island, and return to Kingston on the Monday or Tuesday. I thought it important that my presence was felt, and it gave me firsthand knowledge of what was happening, how people were preparing, what the mood was.

I did quite a bit of troubleshooting along the way. I drew on my ability to make quick decisions with limited information, but knowing that I had a strong foundation of preparation and experience to effectively navigate this complex and uncertain situation. I knew I had to prioritize clear communication, collaboration, and adaptability in responding to the rapidly evolving situation. Civil servants, including public health workers, tend to be inflexible when it comes to rules. They go exactly by the budget and the instructions. By being on site, I realized that I had to use my authority to change rules on the spot, having read the situation and identifying when the rules were hampering the vaccination process.

When I got to Falmouth, Trelawny, on Saturday shortly after noon, there were few people at the vaccination site. We strategized and called the taxi drivers' association head for the area to rally people to come out. At the Montego Bay Convention Centre, there was a crowd, in long lines. We bused in tourism workers to take on the non-medical roles to free up the nurses. I called the head of the BPO association, Gloria Henry, and she agreed to get BPO workers bused in the next day. When I got to Savanna la Mar, my last stop that day, as the crowd diminished, the WRHA chairman and I called around to get more people to the site. On Sunday, the PM called and suggested we invite the journalists to come out. They did, had good experiences, and shared on their social media platforms. On Monday, when I arrived in Southfield, St. Elizabeth, there was a crowd and people waiting in the hot sun. On the spot, I ordered two more tents, rented two hundred chairs, and a private sector leader from the area brought in dozens of cases of water. More vaccinators were brought in to the site.

It was like an election, but without the politics. It felt like a carnival, though maybe not quite as festive.

People were prepared to wait and didn't fuss. This is unusual for Jamaicans. In many locations the JDF was there. Jamaicans respect the army uniform, so that helped. The public health nurses were courteous, and the quality of service was good.

On Monday morning, word got out that the vaccines were going to expire the next day at midnight. Emily Shields (a popular radio personality) tweeted it as "breaking news," and the tweet blew up. The CMO went on Cliff Hughes's programme and calmly explained, in her inimitable way, what expiration dates meant and why the vaccines were perfectly safe and would be safe even after the expiration date. We had anticipated this would happen, and the CMO was prepared. We watched for what the reaction would be. This revelation could either undermine the blitz, and the vaccines would not get administered, or it could spur people to get jabbed while they had the chance.

That is when the blitz became a blast. I didn't go to cabinet that day, as I was still on the road. The overwhelming response, as seen and transmitted over social media, was "Let's go!" People of all ages, especially young people whose turn to be vaccinated wouldn't have come for several months, flooded the vaccination centres that Monday. I went to the Arena on Monday evening and then up to the UWI. Both had extended their hours, and they were buzzing. I felt like I was in an action movie.

At the end of Monday, I checked the numbers. We were going to use all seventy-five thousand doses. We were on our way to accomplishing what many people thought impossible, what we ourselves weren't convinced we could do.

By Tuesday, the increased momentum led to a crescendo, and sites across the island were oversubscribed. I missed Parliament as I was in the field in Kingston and St. Andrew, and that was a good decision. People didn't want to miss out. MPs who hadn't sent their people in before were now eager to be a part of the excitement and get their constituents vaccinated. On Tuesday afternoon, several MPs sent buses full of people to the arena. By this time, all seventy-five thousand doses had been administered. I was there, and after a quick discussion with the CMO and the PS, we sent for eight thousand more doses from our precious stores.

It was a success, but there were instances that bordered on chaos. The rush and the change to the priority group policy made the vaccination programme seem disorganized. The original sequence of priority groups was put on hold as anyone who came received a vaccine; that system would have to be reinstated. The election approach worked in some cases, but the notice was short, and not everyone could manage that, and so some who should have gotten vaccinated didn't. It was like a roller coaster, exhilarating but also scary.

It was one of the few wins of the pandemic that we could see and feel in real time. It worked because we recalibrated as we went along. The teams were given authority to be flexible and adjust as they deemed necessary. The achievement created hope, and the vaccine became something aspirational. The public health teams across the country had shown resilience and commitment in the face of an extraordinary situation. By Tuesday night, they were operating on fumes, and we suspended vaccinations for the rest of the week and the following weekend.

Was this what it would take to get Jamaicans vaccinated? This was not sustainable, just as it wasn't possible to continue testing every arriving passenger at the airport.

We couldn't have known it then, but the difficulties we later faced would make the blitz seem easy.

Post-blitz was a time to pause and reflect. The way we were reporting the numbers and trends had become boring, mundane, and routine and was no longer having an impact. We had been at this for over a year. People had become numb to the same statistics over and over. We needed to shift to something more impactful. In a crisis, it is important to find new and effective ways to present data and information. One must continue to prioritize clear and concise communication to ensure that important information is conveyed accurately and efficiently and recognize the importance of staying flexible. It was time to adapt our approach to information sharing. I asked epidemiology to pivot, to change the way the reports are done. In the first instance, I asked them to compare the second surge to the first.

The data that we shared with the public was illustrative: there were almost four times as many cases in the peak week of the second surge as there were in the first surge. In the first surge's peak week, there were 1,154 cases compared to 4,082 in the second surge's peak week. This translated to the death of some thirty-one persons in the first peak week and fifty-nine in the second. In the first peak week, bed occupancy for confirmed and suspected COVID-19 cases went up to 309, and 716 in the peak week of the second surge.

Presented this way, it was clear how much worse this surge was than the first. The intention was that the public would better appreciate the consequences of reduced movement restrictions and the importance of following the protocols and guidelines. It was unavoidably clear: the pandemic was with us more than ever, and it was getting worse.

Then there was the vaccine shortage, which was proving more of a challenge than we had anticipated. After the blitz, we went back to priority groups as we sought to administer vaccines to those who most needed them first. WHO was moving slowly on approving the vaccines that we thought they would approve. India was in a crisis of its own second wave, with thousands of people dying daily; they stopped exports of the AstraZeneca vaccine to the rest of the world. They were the largest manufacturer of vaccines in the world and had been expected to be the supplier of vaccines to the developing world.

A few cases of post-vaccine blood clots added another layer of chaos, and some countries paused their usage. The reporting of those incidents was perceived by some as skewed and part of the competition between the vaccine manufacturers. The veteran broadcaster Michael Sharpe, a much-loved and popular media personality, was vaccinated in the blitz and died shortly. His death was not caused by the vaccine, but it fueled the anti-vaxxers. Threats were made against the nurse who vaccinated him. Information and misinformation abounded. It was hard to know what to believe.

The virus never stopped changing, and we had no choice but to keep up. We faced the prospect that a low level of vaccination would lead to the development of more variants. But we couldn't say with any certainty the extent of variant strains in the population. The samples were being tested by CARPHA, who had been slow in returning the results. Creating our own testing capacity for variants meant yet another investment in expensive equipment and technology.

The question of whether vaccinated persons were entitled to more freedoms than the non-vaccinated began to surface. The tourism sector began to argue for allowing vaccinated people, tourists and business travelers, more freedom to enter the country. The Bahamas said it saw no need for a test or quarantine for fully vaccinated travelers. It would have implications for restoring normality to the economy, but it would be a logistical challenge, on top of all the other logistical challenges we were already having difficulty meeting with our limited capacity. The question would surely gain strength when more people got vaccinated in Jamaica and in our major tourism markets.

By the end of April, we were finally starting to see the results of the lockdown measures. We were at the lowest positivity rate, 21 percent, since the start of 2021. Trinidad and Tobago, on the other hand, went into a three-week lockdown. Their borders were closed, but the Brazilian variant had gotten in, apparently via illegal migrants crossing over from Venezuela by boat, and was spreading quickly.

I wondered if Jamaicans realized how much more freedom we had than so many others. They hadn't opened their borders since the pandemic started over a year before. Non-nationals could not enter the country, and nationals could not leave. For the few who received exceptions to enter or exit, there were few flights out or in. The question was this: was it worth it to have had such stringent restrictions, which still had not kept the virus out? At least part of the answer was that with an infectious virus like COVID-19, where human beings are the vector, in an island with unpoliced coastal borders, preventing its entry and spread was almost impossible.

As the infection and positivity rate went down, the pressure to ease restrictions increased. After presenting the data on how much worse our second surge was to our first, we projected how much worse a third surge might be compared to the second. The third wave projections would see as many as 10,700 cases, 180 deaths, and 1,900 hospitalisations for confirmed and suspected cases—all in a single week. A third wave would have us overwhelmed, as India had been, with people dying on the streets, and the Ganges River engorged with corpses. We used this to try to convince people to get vaccinated. It didn't seem to have an effect.

We had confirmed which of the variants were in Jamaica. CARPHA had finally sent results from a batch of samples we had sent. Of the ten usable samples, seven were found to have the UK variant, a highly transmissible strain. There was no South African variant and no Brazilian variant. This was good news and bad news. While our numbers were trending down, we were not at a level where we could be comfortable, and the presence of a highly transmissible strain in the population put us at further risk.

At that particular point, the prospects for Jamaica getting all the vaccines that we needed were dim. The US announced they would share 60 million vaccines with the rest of the world. Who would get them had not yet been made public. We would have bought vaccines from them if we could have, especially the AstraZeneca stocks which they had not used and were in storage, certainly with an expiry date approaching. Supplies were unpredictable. Down payments had been made on orders that weren't filled. Delivery date promises were not met. It was impossible for us to plan. On May 30, 2021, we received a second allocation of 55,200 AstraZeneca from COVAX; 40,000 of those were for the blitz recipients to get their second dose, and the remainder for the over-sixty and other priority groups. African Platform was unable to deliver on their commitments. Other avenues were extremely expensive, as high as US$37 a dose. Brokers began to enter the market.

Sourcing vaccines was only one of the concerns as we headed into month fifteen. The economic fallout was evident; despite optimism about a rebound; from what I could see, it wasn't realistic. The impact on children and their education were beginning to present themselves. The toll on people's mental health became apparent. And we anticipated a third wave.

State of Nature |

On May 2, 2021, the Sunday *Gleaner* published an op-ed I wrote. They titled it "COVID-19 and vaccine bundling—when rules do not apply," though my original title for the piece was "Vaccine Nationalism and the State of Nature."

There is a discomfiting contrast between developed and developing countries with regard to vaccines. The former is far advanced in administering vaccines to its population, and the latter are, for the most part, struggling to source them. Up to 40 percent of the population in the developed world has received at least a first dose of the vaccine, while developing countries have only been able to inoculate under seven percent of their population. The World Health Organization's appeals to give greater consideration to smaller and poorer countries have yielded no response.

This disparity threatens the effectiveness of vaccines, which are the most critical response we have to the pandemic. It is also a potential threat to global security and our collective well-being. Despite this, wealthy countries and some pharmaceutical companies are operating by the rules of the jungle despite the WHO's futile attempt to introduce some order and equity. Indeed, we seem to be moving towards a Hobbesian state of nature, where there is a disregard for any notion of the greater good, and it's every country for itself.

Dangers of Self-interest

In this state of nature, where competition over scarce resources heightens the potential for conflict, the priorities become safeguarding one's self-interest and exercising power towards that goal. Vaccines are the scarce resource in a context not only of high demand and limited supply, but of desperation—where the vaccines are a lifeline for countries' economic survival. The wealthier countries have seemingly become blinded to the reality that in a globalised world, individualistic approaches and the rules of the jungle are likely to produce conflict and create divisions between countries.

Hoarding vaccines, and failing to proactively ensure that developing countries are also vaccinating their population, will prolong the pandemic and move those countries dangerously closer to that state of nature.

Further, new strains of COVID-19, such as the so-called Indian, Brazilian, and UK strains, have already affected some countries' vaccination programmes, having rendered some of the vaccines ineffective. It is thus clear that even if wealthier countries are able to sufficiently protect their own population, the virus will continue to spread and to mutate.

COVAX

COVAX, the global vaccine-sharing initiative, was created so that developing countries would have access to vaccines in recognition of the fact that without this kind of a pooling of resources, they would be left in the unvaccinated dark. In addition to an attempt to advance global equity in vaccine access, it was also a practical response to ensuring that all people would be vaccinated as per their slogan: "no one is safe, unless everyone is safe".

However, COVAX has only been able to deliver a fifth of what was promised and expected to just over 100 countries. Jamaica's allotment from COVAX so far is approximately 69,000 doses, well below the two hundred and fifty doses promised by now. COVAX has been unable to fulfil its commitments as a direct result of wealthier countries' actions, including export bans on vaccines and raw materials, which have effectively undermined the facility. The knock-on effect of preventing the export of raw material— as well as India's own struggles to contain the spread of the virus has been to curtail India's initial efforts to assist others through vaccine diplomacy.

Wealthy countries have purchased vaccines in large quantities—up to four times what is required to inoculate their population. Hoarding has become normalised, and supply shortages have worsened as a result. At the same time, there is market manipulation by some pharmaceutical companies, whose naked profit-seeking behaviour is tantamount to exploitation. Among their practices is to set minimum -order quantities, even if those are in excess of the populations of the purchasing country, at prices multiple times the cost of production. The law of the jungle is at work. Meanwhile, the rest of us developing countries must contend with the ongoing effects of the pandemic and the threat of more variant strains.

Global Leadership

We are witnessing—and experiencing—a void in global leadership, and in this pandemic, that void has potentially devastating implications for developing countries.

The pandemic presents a moment to rethink global leadership. States' actions can either weaken international organisations such as the WHO, or they can provide the support that would signal these organisations' critical role in seeing the world through this crisis. In a global arena where large, developed countries' purchasing power threatens to undermine developing countries' prospects for recovering from the pandemic, those organisations can exercise the necessary moral authority to curtail those selfish actions. There have already been calls for the WTO to waive intellectual property rights for vaccine development. The support of the entire international community would help to advance these efforts and initiate other collective strategies.

The Group of Seven committed US$4.3 billion towards an equitable roll-out of the tests, treatments, and vaccines. Without freeing up the supply chains and the raw materials, this commendable contribution could prove difficult in achieving its goal in a timely manner. The US's return to the WHO is welcome, and their recent announcement to distribute vaccines to other countries is also welcome, but not sufficient. The export restrictions, invoked under the Defense Production Act, should be lifted.

Developing countries need vaccines. They need them so that their own economies can recover from the pandemic and so that the world can move towards herd immunity. As each country endeavours to vaccinate its people, the fact that national vaccination programmes' success depends on all countries' vaccination success has to be at the forefront of global leadership. Collective interest, in the context of COVID-19, is not just an ideal, not just a nice concept, it is what will keep the entire world from disintegrating into barbarity and chaos.

Sectoral |

I presented my contribution to the sectoral debate on May 19, 2021. I wanted to give a speech that wasn't only about the pandemic, and I wanted it to be hopeful and forward-looking. I wanted to shift the narrative from the negativity of the pandemic and try, even with the virus still spreading and a vaccine shortage, to highlight hope and resilience. Health had led all the national decisions for the past year, and as the representative of public health among the decision-makers, I had been at the forefront of almost every consideration and debate, and received all the praise and vilification that came with that.

The title and theme of the presentation were, "Hope: Building Back Stronger," the building back referring to what had been lost in the pandemic.

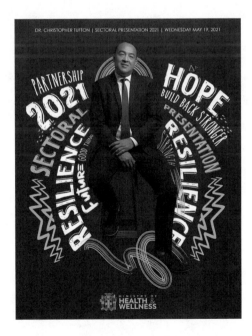

The pandemic was, as to be expected again, the central theme of the speech, but I was determined to include other areas of the ministry's work, activities, and projects that had been forgotten about or overlooked. I thought it was important that we not allow the pandemic to be the only thing we talked about. I also wanted to use the opportunity to present the positive aspects of the pandemic, how the system had been strengthened and made more resilient, how more healthcare workers had been hired, how the number of ICU beds had doubled. These were all forward steps that would continue to redound to our benefit after the pandemic was over, though at that time when that would happen was anyone's best guess. I returned to my pre-COVID-19 themes of personal responsibility to pursue a better quality of life, through health-seeking behaviours and lifestyle choices.

(excerpts from 2021 sectoral)

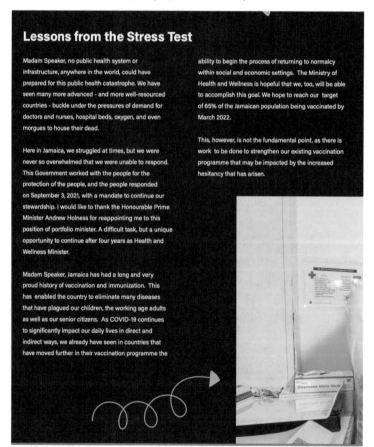

Lessons from the Stress Test

Madam Speaker, no public health system or infrastructure, anywhere in the world, could have prepared for this public health catastrophe. We have seen many more advanced - and more well-resourced countries - buckle under the pressures of demand for doctors and nurses, hospital beds, oxygen, and even morgues to house their dead.

Here in Jamaica, we struggled at times, but we were never so overwhelmed that we were unable to respond. This Government worked with the people for the protection of the people, and the people responded on September 3, 2021, with a mandate to continue our stewardship. I would like to thank the Honourable Prime Minister Andrew Holness for reappointing me to this position of portfolio minister. A difficult task, but a unique opportunity to continue after four years as Health and Wellness Minister.

Madam Speaker, Jamaica has had a long and very proud history of vaccination and immunization. This has enabled the country to eliminate many diseases that have plagued our children, the working age adults as well as our senior citizens. As COVID-19 continues to significantly impact our daily lives in direct and indirect ways, we already have seen in countries that have moved further in their vaccination programme the

ability to begin the process of returning to normalcy within social and economic settings. The Ministry of Health and Wellness is hopeful that we, too, will be able to accomplish this goal. We hope to reach our target of 65% of the Jamaican population being vaccinated by March 2022.

This, however, is not the fundamental point, as there is work to be done to strengthen our existing vaccination programme that may be impacted by the increased hesitancy that has arisen.

Two Jamaicas |

Jamaica's entertainment sector was among the hardest hit by the pandemic. Stage shows, dances, parties, round robins, and cookouts had been banned since March 2020 as part of the government's measures to stem the spread of the pandemic. Even when curfews were extended and gathering limits were increased, the sector was still dormant because of other rules prohibiting them from operating. Stakeholders from that sector had been restive, persistently lobbying to get some concession to alleviate their situation. Whereas other sectors had had some relief, such as the restaurant sector with the development of the ENDS delivery app, the entertainment sector had no such intervention.

At the same time, there had been remarkably little commentary about freedom of movement and quarantine for tourists. Apart from the rumblings about inequality regarding rules for tourists (and, to a lesser extent, business visitors) in the early days of the border reopening, there had been no complaints about what tourists could do versus the rules for Jamaicans. Tourists on the north coast could move about within the "resilient corridor" while it wasn't clear if Jamaicans could do so, but no one seemed to notice.

So, when an overseas (US) event promoter brought hundreds of party-goers to Jamaica to celebrate Mocha Fest, whose tag line was "The Wildest Urban Festival on Earth," it was problematic. Mocha Fest was a five-day, eight-party event, from May 24 to 31, 2021. Each party was to take place at a different location. It was an annual event over the US Memorial Day holiday weekend, and it had been staged for the previous seven years, but was cancelled in 2020.

It came to the public's attention on Day 3, when an event at Rick's Cafe in Negril was closed down by the police for violating the number of people that could be in one place. It soon came to light that the event had been widely advertised on the festival's website and social media pages, offering hotel packages and excursions and advising guests to book early. The event also appeared on the Jamaica Tourist Board's "Visit Jamaica" website (the entire events page was removed when the uproar began), and promotional material for Mocha Fest carried the Tourist Board's logo.

It was another instance that COVID-19 brought about where Jamaicans (especially those active on social media) perceived that there was inequality in how the rules were applied. The familiar refrain of "two Jamaicas" was heard. That phrase usually refers to the differences in the worlds of the country's haves and the have-nots, or to the notion that different rules are applied depending on a person's status in the society. Now, the two Jamaicas concept had a new application: COVID-19 rules for tourists and different rules for Jamaicans in their own country.[73]

The Mocha Fest debacle spurred forward movement on reopening the entertainment industry. It also represented a dilution of the government's authority and ability to enforce restrictions. The numbers were trending down, and the calls from the sector could no longer be ignored. The public health caution remained: all events where large numbers of people were gathered and were in close proximity could result in increased risk of exposure to COVID-19 to the participants. Regardless of the positivity rate, once the virus was present, several people mingling in a party-like setting provided the ideal conditions for the virus to spread widely. But the horse was already out the gate, and all public health could do was prepare for the fallout.

By June 2021, Month 15 of the pandemic, contracting COVID-19 was no longer remarkable. One year before, it was shameful, stigmatized. Now it was commonplace. One of my sons contracted it, apparently from someone he played football with in the afternoons. He wasn't severely ill, and no one else in the household tested positive. He

---

[73] "As Tourists Party, Citizens Under COVID Lockdown Ask: Are There Two Jamaicas?" *Global Voices*, May 29, 2021, https://globalvoices.org/2021/05/29/as-tourists-party-citizens-under-covid-lockdown-ask-are-there-two-jamaicas/.

isolated at home and recovered. I was reminded of how remarkable it was that I hadn't caught the virus, at least not that I had known.

We were still in remission from the second wave. Curfews and other movement restrictions remained. New positives were low, less than a hundred per day. (This perspective that "low" was one hundred was such a drastic difference from the days when one hundred was an alarming high.) But testing was not being done as assiduously, so the absolute was not reliable. The Delta variant , what was previously called the UK variant (though it originated in India), loomed. The United Kingdom had delayed its reopening by a month because of its spread. This variant was more contagious and therefore spread faster. While most vaccines were effective against serious illness from the variant, none could prevent its transmission.

By then, we had a new vaccine problem on our hands: insufficient supply of AstraZeneca to administer second doses to those who had gotten a first dose in the blitz. We frantically tried to source from all over. Between Foreign Affairs Minister, Kamina Johnson-Smith, NHF Chair Howard Mitchell, and myself, we worked the phones, with prime ministers, presidents, other health ministers, technocrats, and heads of international organizations. Lots of promises were made, but few delivered. A Caribbean neighbour secretly sent us a few spare they had, though they ought to have returned any unused vaccines to COVAX.

People were angry and disappointed, and rightfully so. This failure to provide second doses could result in people losing trust in the system and slowing the vaccine take-up momentum. In addition, it lowered the prospects of us successfully reducing vaccine hesitancy. It was another reminder that nothing in this pandemic was ever assured. So much uncertainty existed, from one moment to another. One day you're up, the next one you're down. It was impossible to predict and impractical to rely on promises. We had no idea when the pandemic would end or what to expect even in the days and weeks directly ahead of us.

Our efforts to secure second doses for the blitz eventually succeeded. Mexico sent sixty-five thousand doses of AstraZeneca on a Mexican Air Force jet. Again, there was a ceremonious reception at the airport, a diplomatic coup for the Mexicans. The US still promised to make millions of vaccines available to other countries. If we could get a million vaccines within the next month or two, it might prevent a deadlier third wave than the one we were expecting. But that much-anticipated donation from the US was held up by regional and bilateral politics.

The positive development of having the doses available was countered by disorganization on the ministry's side. The appointment system wasn't working. Vaccination sites were overrun. People with appointments were not getting through. Again, avoidable problems were causing frustration.

Adding to the flow of news I would rather have not had, a "lab leak theory" investigation was ordered by US President Biden. My primary thought was this would strengthen the conspiracy theorists and further undermine vaccine take-up. This was tantamount to giving the anti-vax movement fodder to continue to undermine the attempts at controlling the pandemic. Nothing significant was uncovered from that investigation.

Did it matter where the virus originated? I revisited this question often. Knowing if it had come from a lab, it wouldn't change anything that had happened, nor the situation we found ourselves in now. And the implications of this catastrophe having been man-made were overwhelming.

In the midst of the ongoing uncertainty of the pandemic, there was one thing I could count on: no matter what was done, what decision was taken, what measure was imposed or lifted, there would always be detractors.

Doctors were unhappy. Just as the government was relaxing measures that would lead to more work and risk for them, they were restive.

They were dissatisfied with their gratuity agreement, their contract tenure, and the 147 doctors who needed jobs. On this issue, it was not entirely on the government or public health sector. UWI had been training more doctors since they had expanded their capacity, who they assumed would be hired by the government. There was a sense of entitlement to getting a public sector job that had set in over time.

I coped with the pressure with physical activity. I had progressed in my swimming lessons from breaststroke to freestyle. Swimming became the most relaxing activity I engaged in. It was meditative. I felt free in the water, especially now that I could move through it with my newfound swimming skills. I even felt emotionally lighter. It was the closest I came to feeling worry- and problem-free. I was still running, cycling, and strength-training. My exercise routine was saving me from physical and mental collapse.

I contemplated a theory: COVID-19 had forced us to restructure our lives, and it wasn't all to our detriment. In fact, some of it was a better way to live. We were earlier to bed and earlier to rise. Starting and leaving an event, a bar, or a gathering earlier than we used to wasn't a bad thing. Road accidents were down. Accident and emergency numbers were down. Hospitalisations were down (though a lot of elective surgery was cancelled).

I was going day by day, but I knew I was managing relatively well. Many others were fatigued and depressed. Could I do anything about that? Was that something I should concern myself with? I considered my duty at that moment was to give succour. I wanted to impart a renewed sense of hope for the future and show how we were going to get there, as individuals, as communities, and as a country. I wanted to advance a perspective that showed how resilient we have been that despite the deaths and the economic fallout, Jamaica could be proud of not having had a disastrous experience, at least up to that point.

I wanted to bring about a reset of the national state of mind. But the third wave on the horizon came with the strictest containment measures ever. A reset would have to wait.

Dream Weekend |

July 2021. Seventeen months. This was reopening month. We were at the low end of the "medium level of spread" spectrum. We saw a sustained decrease in the positivity rate since the peak of 39 percent four months earlier. Curfews were shortened to 11:00 pm. The importance of events such as parties and festivals in supporting the social aspects of health and well-being were being recognized. Gathering restrictions were loosened. Permission was given for entertainment events.

We reopened knowing a third wave was heading our way. The Delta variant was surely in Jamaica. It had ravaged India and done damage in the UK. The reopening made it affecting us more inevitable, as not only would people be moving about and gathering, but people would be traveling to the island as well. We didn't have a high enough vaccination rate to make any meaningful difference in what was certain to happen. I didn't push back against the decision to reopen, but I did instruct the ministry to prepare for that third wave we knew would come. It wasn't a risk, it was a guarantee, and I made this clear. We would have to retreat in preparation to advance.

The debate over reopening was sustained. On one side was the belief that we couldn't stay closed any longer, that the economic and social costs now outweighed the public health costs, that people's mental and psychosocial well-being had to be prioritized, that the country was near boiling point. As vocal and influential as one subset of the country had been (those pushing for reopening), there was another clamorous group that was bitter, and they made their concerns known. The other side, pushed heavily by influential media personalities and social media voices, was critical: "Too much, too soon," they repeated.

It was a no-win situation. The crisis brought on by the pandemic required that at any given time, any policy had to aim towards a greater good, not an absolute good. An absolute good just did not exist. And by this time, we, the government, accepted we would never please everybody, and that in fact we had lost ground in trying to please everybody.

The health ministry was tasked to develop protocols and guidelines for a "safe reopening." There was a proposal for a phased approach, where things would open up more gradually, depending on the transmission rate, cap the number of people allowed at an event to one hundred, and hold back on allowing large entertainment events. The limit was set to two hundred. The rule was there should be a minimum of two trained COVID-19 monitors/marshals for every fifty persons at the venue. The proposed guidelines were that entertainment venues and activities should be rigorously monitored by the promoter/manager of the event and by the monitors/marshals (under the purview of the Ministry of Local Government and Community Development) to ensure compliance with the measures.

Whether those rules and guidelines were ever implemented is unknown. The opening of the entertainment sector was short-lived. A surge just a few weeks after, what would be our third and deadliest wave of the entire pandemic, would suggest that even if they were implemented, they were ineffective.

Once movement restrictions were lifted, people throughout the island not only resumed a semblance of pre-COVID-19 normal life, but there was also a pent up desire to be out and socialize, whether at parties or at church.

Dream Weekend was a five-day, back-to-back party experience staged every year in Negril over the Emancipendence weekend (Emancipation Day August 1 and Independence Day August 6). It had not happened in 2020, and the timing of the reopening was perfect for this event to resume. There were several such events all over the island, legal and illegal, where people gyrated whether with the holy spirit or from the effects of spirits. Most were not staged by such a well-recognized brand; some were simply street dances, some were community round robins, but all offered Jamaicans some much-longed-for fun and excitement.

Dream Weekend can't be said to have caused the surge, but with the videos from the event showing hundreds of mask-less people drinking, dancing, in swimming pools, and making merry with not even six inches between them, that event came to symbolize it. There were several such events all over the island. With the Delta variant , it didn't take a super-spreader event to kick off a surge. With such an exponential increase in people's contact with one another, the surge was going to happen.

The name Dream Weekend was also symbolic of us having unrealistic dreams of normality without consequence—that we could think we could make rules such as having COVID-19 marshals at parties keeping people six feet apart, and events requiring vaccination cards or COVID-19 tests, and that those rules would make a difference. We were definitely dreaming.

The dreaming extended beyond parties and events. I did a double take at the *Gleaner* front page on August 17, 2021. There was a large photo the Carnival Sunshine, the first cruise ship to come to Jamaica since March 2020. It had pulled into the Ocho Rios Cruise Terminal in St. Ann the day before. The ship's arrival heralded the cruise industry's return to "normalcy." Ninety-four percent of the passengers, it was said, were vaccinated against the virus. A team from the Ministry of Health and Wellness was there to assist passengers to sanitise their hands and conduct temperature checks. We were resuming an activity that was a known facilitator of the spread of COVID-19, amidst several valid questions about the sustainability and real value of that activity beyond COVID-19, and it was being "heralded." It gave me pause.

It was the first sign that we were going to go through this pandemic and not build on the learning that had been forced on us. There would be many more of these signs in the months to come.

Whereas the time between Christmas and the second wave was several weeks, the third wave came quickly on the heels of Emancipendence. On August 19, 2021, the strictest COVID-19 containment measures we had experienced since the beginning of the pandemic were announced. The dreaded third wave that we knew would come had reached us, and it was as bad as was predicted. Seven "no movement" days—in effect, lockdown—were to run over a period of three weeks, and new curfews were imposed. We had never done such extensive movement restrictions before, covering the following Sunday, Monday, and Tuesday; the Sunday, Monday, and Tuesday after that, and Sunday September 5. New curfew hours were 7:00 pm to 5:00 am, except on Saturdays when the curfew would begin at 6:00 pm. After September 5, the measures would be reviewed, based on what the infection rates were.

Up to this point, seventeen months in, there had been early curfews on Sundays, and a few public holidays that were completely no movement, but this was new. No entertainment events, large or small, were permitted, and there were gathering limits for churches, weddings, and funerals. Nightclubs and "places of amusement" were to be closed, and gyms, restaurants, and bars were ordered to operate at 50 percent capacity. The reopening of schools in September was thrown into doubt. Ultimately, it didn't happen.

The day before the new measures were announced, on August 18, 2021, we had received confirmation that the Delta variant was present in Jamaica. We had sent sixty samples to CARPHA in Trinidad and Tobago, received forty results, and twenty-two were positive for the Delta variant . We were already working with the premise that the variant was in the island; here was the confirmation.

The Delta variant was the most prevalent COVID-19 variant of the pandemic up to that point. It had been reported in over one hundred countries, and was responsible for surges in several countries. Two dozen countries had epidemiological curves that were almost vertical, signaling the meteoric spread of this mutated virus. In the US, the Delta variant accounted for 51 percent of new cases and was driving case and death numbers up across the country, with daily caseloads having increased tenfold between late June and the first two weeks of July, hospitalizations back at February 2021 levels, and death reports having doubled. In the UK, the Delta variant caused a quadrupling of cases in one month and was the cause of 95 percent of new cases. Several other countries had seen surges in cases and deaths and had reimposed restrictions. Jamaica never stood a chance.

The variant was so deadly because early in the infection, when people were most likely to be contagious, it replicated in amounts that were thought to be one thousand times as much as was seen in people infected with other variants, defeating immune defenses in the nose and throat. The major vaccines appeared to be effective against Delta, in preventing severe illness and death, though people still contracted the virus, as the vaccine did not affect transmission. The Delta variant made people sicker than any previous variant, and the unvaccinated were getting sicker than COVID-19-infected people had before.

The Delta variant wasn't the first "variant of concern," as the WHO and technical team referred to them. A variant was considered as such if it was found to have increased transmissibility or brought a detrimental change in COVID-19 epidemiology; was more virulent, was different in how it presented, and therefore meant a decrease in effectiveness of public health and social measures or available diagnostics, vaccines, and therapeutics. These variants were also identified to cause significant community transmission or multiple COVID-19 clusters in multiple countries, with increasing relative prevalence alongside increasing numbers of cases over time or other apparent epidemiological impacts to suggest an emerging risk to global public health.

We knew what to do. If there was one certainty in how this pandemic worked in Jamaica, it was that restricting movement with curfews and lockdowns brought down infection rates. As night follows day. We proved that in the third wave and then later again in the fourth.

Those new, extreme measures had been preceded by measures that brought the short-lived reopening to an end. From an 11:00 pm curfew and gathering limits of two hundred, we had gone back to Mondays to Fridays 7:00 pm to 5:00 am, Saturdays 6:00 pm to 5:00 am, and Sundays 2:00 pm to 5:00 am. Those were supposed to run until August 31, but the infection rate climbed so high so quickly that more extreme measures had to be implemented.

We knew why and how this had happened: the reopening, the Delta variant , and the long holiday, Emancipendence weekend, were a deadly combination.

Every decision comes with consequences. These were the consequences for our decisions.

Morale among the public health team was low. They knew this would happen. They felt that they had made it clear to us as decision-makers what would be the outcome of reopening in the way that it was done. They were over-ruled, and now they would be asked to save the day.

Blame was everywhere. It was "someone's" fault that we had a third wave.

From one corner, it was low vaccination rates: the virus surged because not enough people had taken the vaccine. Mind you, when we couldn't get vaccines and demand exceeded supply, we were roundly criticized, though vaccine unavailability was beyond our control. Now we had them, and people weren't getting vaccinated. The low take-up was somehow the government's fault. This, of course, was wrong in so many ways, not least that the vaccines did not prevent transmission. They reduced the severity of the illness once it was contracted, but would only slow transmission (because the ill person would have a lower viral load) if it had any effect at all. There would have been less illness and fewer deaths. So the surge would likely still have happened, but it would probably not have had such terrible outcomes.

From another corner: we opened up too fast and too soon. This line of argument conveniently left out that the opening happened in the context of a powder keg about to explode. Either the government relaxed the restrictions, or people would break them anyway, and it would be chaos.

Everyone was frustrated and angry. The surge meant that school could not reopen in September. It was a blow to the children, their parents, and teachers who had struggled with remote schooling for over a year and who were anxious to get back to in-person classes. The studies worldwide, and the preliminary data from Jamaica, suggested that learning losses were high and that the lost year and a half of learning would have detrimental effects on those children's mental health, life prospects, and on the country's development as a whole. My concerns about the economic fallout and the mental health consequences of the pandemic were now added to by a preoccupation about children, education, and the country's future.

The reopening was one step forward, and now we were taking two steps back. It felt like the pandemic would never end.

Irony |

The vaccine shortage problem was at least resolved. Between vaccine diplomacy—what other countries had gifted us—and our own procurement efforts, we had enough for the entire population. The arrival of a shipment of the Pfizer vaccine, the first of three batches donated by the United States, ought to have signaled good news for children going back to school, as this vaccine was safe for children twelve years old and up. But the surge got there first.

But we were having problems with delivering the vaccines to the people who wanted them. The logistical demands of such a major undertaking had gotten the better of the ministry's limited capacity. Vaccination sites were crowded with long lines, and people were being turned away. The rollout needed to be revamped at several levels. Even still, that could not be said to have caused the low vaccine rates we were experiencing.

And then another irony: we were faced with the prospect of having too many vaccines. Because many of the orders we had placed were delayed in being fulfilled, we now had an excess supply, and most of the donated vaccines were set to expire within a few months. In some cases, the donated vaccines were in excess of what those countries needed, and they had dumped them on us since they were about to expire on them. Yes, we needed them, and while we were grateful, it also put us under pressure. At the rate we were going, we could not use them all up. After being desperate for vaccines, subjected to unmet expectations from other countries who we thought would look out for us, here we were with excess about-to-expire vaccines and the galling prospect of having to dump them ourselves.

We began to tackle the low take-up challenge. The National Health Fund chairman commissioned a snap poll. A team went out in the streets of Mandeville and Christiana one Saturday morning (market day) and ascertained the reasons for the low take-up. The responses were thought-provoking:

- Too many negatives about the vaccine

- Too many people getting sick after being vaccinated

- Don't know what's in the vaccine

- Still awaiting more information

- Scared of symptoms I'll have (side effects)

- Doesn't stop you from contracting the virus

- It's ready too quick

- Don't trust the vaccine or the government

- People are dying either way

- Not sure if the virus is even real

- Fear of injection

It didn't help when reports of "breakthrough" infections began to surface—people who had been vaccinated but who had tested positive for COVID-19. Why take the vaccine when it doesn't prevent catching the virus? It was never meant to prevent transmission or immunize someone from contracting COVID-19. The vaccines produced antibodies in the blood that prevented the coronavirus from taking root in those organs, but they could not prevent infection. What vaccines could do was prevent hospitalization and death and the worst outcomes of infection, such as damage to the lungs and other organs. In our push to encourage people to get vaccinated, we had not emphasized that, and that nuance had been lost. Now it was being interpreted as a bait and switch.

CAPRI later did a study on vaccine hesitancy that delved a bit deeper. Some of the results were surprising.[74] When the survey was done in mid-2021, Jamaica's vaccination rate was the second lowest in the Caribbean region. It was clear from then that we would not reach the goal of vaccinating 65 percent of the population by March 31, 2022. (We never did. We got to around 27 percent, not including boosters.) The typical profile of the vaccine-hesitant Jamaican, according to the study, was a young, low-income person, more likely male than female, but not significantly so, who did not finish primary school, was not religious, was not complacent, but was risk averse, and who did not trust the government or the vaccine.

Another finding: politicians should not be the face of vaccination campaigns, as they were the least likely to be able to convince a vaccine-hesitant person to get inoculated. Much of what we had to promote vaccination, however, had done just that. When I saw that finding, I recognized it was obvious. But it was also obvious that we were way past that stage. The findings would have been useful six months before, perhaps.

Those findings turned out to be academic. They came too late for the evidence to be useful. By the time the CAPRI study came out in January 2022, we were in a fourth wave, and Jamaicans' interest in COVID-19 vaccines had plummeted to almost zero.

---

[74] "Long Shot: Aiming to Reduce Vaccine Hesitancy."

Time Come |

The impact was as bad as the epidemiological modeling predicted. Higher infection rates, more serious illness, and more hospitalizations and deaths than the second wave. We registered one thousand new cases a day consistently, and the positivity rate was over 50 percent, which we considered lower than it actually was, due to underreporting.

At this point, I pushed for a tactical shift in the communications strategy. People needed to see the reality of COVID-19. I decided to portray the hospitals in distress. I got footage of a hospital porter dressed in full protective gear pushing what seemed to be a dead body on a gurney, with an ominous voiceover narrating the numbers of people sick and dying. Prominent journalist Dionne Jackson Miller was allowed access to the Savanna-la-Mar Hospital. She gave a report about how crowded it was, which shocked many people. The intention was to administer shock therapy to the country to say, "People are dying, and your chances of survival are low if you get to the ICU, indeed if you get a bed at all. If you get vaccinated, you can avoid this fate."

I had another goal in this new approach: to give the nurses a voice. They were frustrated by many things, including a drawn-out wage negotiation with the government, through the Ministry of Finance. About one thousand nurses formed their own caucus, apart from the Nurses Association of Jamaica (NAJ, the lead negotiator for the nurses). They formed WhatsApp chat groups where they communicated and strategized. They seized an opportunity when the prime minister made an innocuous comment at a media briefing that there would be no special priority groups of persons who would have access to COVID-19 treatment (given the shortage of beds). They either took the comment out of context or deliberately used it as a red herring. Either way, that was their basis for taking industrial action.

I mooted a one-off payment to the nurses to ease tensions and show appreciation for their efforts. That eventually found its way into the wage negotiations.

Healthcare workers were demoralized as they had to carry the burden of this third wave that they also had seen coming. The only way to overcome the issue of losing the healthcare workers, given the wage issues, would be to give them recognition and a voice, and to let them be seen and heard and feel seen and heard. It may have been a maverick approach to try to keep them motivated, but I believe it helped to relieve some of the pent-up tension.

Together, with the solemn messages to the public, I very well understood it was pursuing a negative approach, which governments tend not to do. There were those in government who were loath to deliberately instill fear in people, and some didn't like it. I thought it worked to jolt people out of complacency (though that was my own perception, I had no metric to prove it.)

If I hadn't scared people enough with the gloomy ads, then something truly scary happened: at the height of our worst wave of COVID-19, we had another oxygen shortage.

Haven't we been through this already? I asked. I knew the answer, of course. In March, we had an oxygen shortage when Jamaica's sole supplier of oxygen ran into supply chain issues. Following that, they had fulfilled their promise to invest in capital equipment to manufacture more oxygen and had been keeping up with the increased demand since the pandemic, oftentimes working around the clock to get oxygen to hospitals. Now a video circulated on social media of a woman in desperate need of oxygen. It was distressing, and scarier than anything I could have put in an ad.

IGL, the only supplier of medical oxygen on the island, had a contract with the government which was regularly renegotiated and renewed. At the last contract renewal, IGL had requested a 26 to 27 percent rate increase, which the MOHW deemed unreasonable. We considered exploring what other oxygen supply options there might be, not only because of this high rate increase, but also given the reasonable concern of being over-reliant on one supplier. This meant that a new contract had not been signed. The traditional and known custom is that until a contract is renewed or replaced, the terms of the pre-existing contract apply, and IGL was being compensated according to the terms of the expired contract.

IGL was now out of oxygen, because, they said, the demand was greater than they were told it would be, worldwide demand had increased, and they weren't able to source any to import. They put out a press release suggesting that the ministry had not given them adequate information, hence they had not anticipated the demand. It was a puzzling release, unnecessary because we were not intending to be antagonistic. IGL had performed well up to that point. If the shortage was due to factors out of their control, that was a problem that had to be worked through. But the press release brought things to the public domain that were neither necessary nor desirable, including the contract negotiations.

What followed was predictable: we were accused of "failing to plan" and thus "planning to fail." It added fodder to those who were critical of the pandemic management and placed myself and the government under even more pressure. Worse, the implication of IGL's press release was a dereliction of duty on our part. I couldn't allow the public health team to be wrongly accused, nor should their confidence be undermined. We had given IGL a projection on the third wave and had the paper trail to prove it. Once again, we were spending time and energy—the PS was up until 3:00 am drafting a response to the IGL statement—on problems that shouldn't have been problems in the first place. We needed the focus to be on solving the public health crisis.

The oxygen shortage was remedied by the Monday, and the worst case scenario of people dying for lack of oxygen did not happen. The idea was floated that for all the stress, the episode may have gotten more people to get vaccinated. The vaccination data wasn't able to confirm that, but it was the anecdotal conclusion. If it were actually so, that it took a crisis of that magnitude to wake people up to what COVID-19 could do to an unvaccinated person, the prospects for increased uptake were indeed dim.

Every time I thought we had hit the lowest point, something else found us at new depths. By now, so many people had died that everyone had either lost a family member, or was one degree separated from someone who had. There was despair all around: those who were mourning lost loved ones; parents grieving the shattered promise of school reopening; business people, large and small, being cut off yet again; and overwhelmed and burnt out healthcare workers.

Everyone was flapping around: "Something has to be done!" they all said.

No one had ever stopped "doing." The crisis had been one of continuous and rapid change, from one week to another. From one day to another, we were faced with new situations, new challenges. And whenever we seemed to be getting it right, some new development would take place, and we were back at the beginning.

A New Vaccine Push |

On September 1, 2021, the movement restriction measures were extended for two more weeks. We were yet to see any improvement in infection rates, hospitalizations, or deaths, but there was a sense that things were normalizing—to the "new normal," that is. We had to continue with the measures if we were going to get a handle on the surge. Six more no-movement days would take us to mid-September. We all hoped that by then we would see some change.

The opposition, People's National Party (PNP), called for my resignation: "Dr. Tufton has repeatedly failed in his handling of the pandemic," they stated. "Eighteen months into the pandemic, the country does not have a proper COVID-19 management plan," and "the oxygen shortage is the latest demonstration of the failure to exercise duty of care." Further, "many of the more than one thousand five hundred deaths could have been prevented had the government put in place proper measures and enhanced the healthcare infrastructure."

The general reaction among Jamaicans: "I of to laugh" (I have to laugh). Not for a second was I concerned by that. They must have thought that the oxygen crisis was a good opening, that it would have weakened me and my standing. But when even the comrades (PNP supporters and members) came out on social media defending me, they must have realized it was a misstep. They couldn't have known this, but they actually did me a favour as some of the pushback towards me by some of my political colleagues got dialed down. I am sure a few, maybe more than a few, would have liked to see the back of me, given how much of an obstacle they saw me as, but when they witnessed the outpouring of public support for me that was awoken by the PNP's call, they saw that I had more currency than they had realized. The quote that says "politics is a strife of interests masquerading as a contest of principles" could not have been truer.[75]

---

[75] Ambrose Bierce, American writer and Civil War veteran.

The more substantive business of the day was the vaccination programme. We had shipments coming in on almost a weekly basis by now, whether donations, from COVAX or the African Platform, or vaccines we had directly purchased. By now, it was clear to all that vaccine hesitancy was far worse than they could have imagined. At the same time, there was a strong belief that getting people vaccinated was our only hope to end the scourge that the pandemic had on the country. An all-day cabinet subcommittee huddle to try to figure out how to change the trajectory led to some new initiatives.

We agreed that the logistical shortcomings were unacceptable. People waiting six hours, oftentimes standing up in the hot sun, would turn people away from getting vaccinated. We would broaden the vaccination channels and expand the outlets to administer the vaccines to the airport, to private contractors, and to community-based organizations and put less emphasis on the centralized sites. There would be multiple channels, all with a protocol and oversight from MOHW. People would have options for where to get a vaccine.

We set out to raise the energy level around vaccination. To that end, the prime minister set out to do an island-wide tour, with a goal of mobilizing and motivating people to get vaccinated. As he put it in Parliament: he went out there to get people to vote, and he would go out there to get people vaccinated. I had always thought this was the most viable approach not only to get people vaccinated but also to attempt to ensure equity in the vaccination process. This was the approach in the original blitz. The plan was for each constituency to hire forty people for four weeks to canvass and bring people out. They would be given shirts and caps with the vaccine message. Sites would be set up close to the population centres. Each MP would get $650,000 to pay workers and mobilize, and they would be provided with transportation. It was an expensive venture, but this was what we thought it would take to move the vaccination rate needle.

The shortage of healthcare workers to administer vaccines would be ameliorated by training private doctors and school nurses, and we would issue a request for proposals (RFP) to private entities to administer vaccines, and we the government would pay them J$1,000 per dose administered. Also costly, but we were pursuing every option. We would embark on a private sector initiative, where medium and large companies would hold in-house drives for their employees and their employees' family members. A vaccine oversight committee was created to take the roll out of the Ministry of Health and Wellness, though the ministry would still participate and play a key role.

I also went back out on the road. The PM went east to St. Thomas; I went west to Hanover. Vaccination sites were open during the lockdowns, and I went to several each day, to observe, motivate the healthcare workers, and maintain the energy around the vaccination drive. A three-day lockdown brings a peculiar mood to the public space. It was otherworldly. We would go from completely empty roads for three days to heavily congested traffic from early on the Wednesday morning as the country scrambled to make up for the time lost.

Our satisfaction that we had sufficient vaccines, however, was interrupted by a shortage of the Pfizer vaccine, which was needed to give the second dose to the twelve to eighteen-year-olds who had received the first dose in August. On September 10, we had to suspend administration of the Pfizer vaccine when the expected second donated shipment from the USA had not arrived. Many Jamaicans preferred Pfizer, which was originally slated only for children, as there was no other approved vaccine for them. We were administering Pfizer to everyone, on the premise that we would have adequate supplies. The thinking was, if people are willing to be vaccinated, and they insist that it be a certain brand, give it to them. But now, the second dose for several tens of thousands of people, including children, was looking iffy. Any lingering hope that schools might reopen for in-person learning was definitively shattered. Frustration and anger spread even further. We eventually got the doses we needed near the end of October, just within the time band for the second dose. Suriname donated 45,630 doses, and 100,620 doses we bought through COVAX.

On September 15, the weekday no-movement days were discontinued, but Sunday remained. An 8:00 pm to 5:00 am curfew was set for weekdays, and 6:00 pm on Saturdays. Those measures were set to run until October 28, 2021. It was put to Jamaica that we weren't "loosening" the measures, but that since there had been congestion especially on public transportation, with the no-movement days, this was a necessary step. Public gathering limits remained at ten, and church services and weddings had limits of twenty people. Public sector workers would continue to work from home. Some grumbled, some accepted it without complaint. There was no way to satisfy everyone in this pandemic. There was no way to prioritize one group's needs or demands over another's. And yet, despite the dissatisfaction, when time came to consider hard data, we actually were not doing badly.

At least once a year, polls are done in Jamaica to measure political leaders' popularity and how much trust citizens have in them and how citizens feel about their performance. These are usually commissioned by a media house which then reports on the findings for the weeks to follow.

"Trust in Tufton at an all-time high." In September 2021, two sets of polls were reported, Blue Dot and Don Anderson, both established, credible pollsters. The Blue Dot polls showed the prime minister and me polling ahead of our cabinet colleagues. That is, the survey said we were the best-performing ministers. PM Holness was considered "the best" by 32 percent of respondents (it was a representative sample), while 25 percent considered me "the best." The numbers for me were higher than in previous polls, suggesting that the regard for me had risen over the pandemic, not fallen. I was also considered the most suitable minister to carry Jamaica through the pandemic. Most gratifying was that my ministry polled better than the national government in the level of trust the Jamaican people have in them managing the COVID-19 pandemic.[76]

Then came the moment that we dreaded: at midnight on September 30, we found ourselves discarding fifty-five thousand expired doses of AstraZeneca that had been donated by the United Kingdom on July

---

[76] "NNN-BlueDot Poll: The Majority of Jamaicans Trust the Health Minister to Manage the COVID-19 Pandemic," *Nationwide 90FM News*, September 7, 2021, https://nationwideradiojm.com/nnn-bluedot-poll-the-majority-of-jamaicans-trust-the-health-minister-to-manage-the-covid-19-pandemic/.

30. We extended hours at vaccination sites to try to use up as many as possible, but the willingness to be vaccinated still just wasn't there. This was a tough one. After all we had been through to get vaccines, that we now had to dump them was galling. There was a time when one missing vial of vaccine was a national crisis.

That question again: who was to blame? In the eyes of the critics, it was the ministry's fault, the government's fault, my fault, even. I refused to accept that, and again, I went maverick and on the offensive. I had a new hashtag, #TimeCome. At the outset of my tenure in the portfolio, I realized and promoted the notion of personal responsibility when it comes to one's health status, so my putting this on the people of Jamaica was in line with what I had been saying all along.

My tweets:

......

Sep. 30th, the last day before expiration of this batch of vaccines there was a rush on sites. Over 17k vaccinated on that day. A week before only 1.5K turned up. Not an issue of sites. The issue is us! #TimeCome

......

.....

The health team delivered 245k of this batch of vaccines in 2months expir. date. Over 40 VAX sites each day, empty @ times- over 25k pass their 8 week due date – where are they? At what point do we speak about personal responsibility? Or say get Vax or else…? #TimeCome

.....

I was fed up with trying to please everybody; by that point, I had accepted it wasn't possible. And that was starting to show.

Here to Stay |

Going to cabinet each Monday was draining. I began to approach a feeling of dread when the time came. I met with the CMO and the PS before cabinet each week to go over their presentations and what their recommendations would be so we would have a pre-game plan. We still made a formidable team, though the initial exhilaration had long worn off. We would spend hours discussing vaccines and other COVID-19 matters, and most of it amounted to an interrogation of me. We debated whether lockdowns work. We knew it was not a long-term solution, but it cauterized the spikes in the short term, and that was important and valuable. Ultimately, I was tasked with finding the balance between the policy-makers and the public health position. Those are days that I do not remember fondly.

To be fair, I also wanted to see the back of COVID-19. There was other important work. The rehabilitation of Cornwall Regional Hospital was, for me, the principal project that the pandemic had stalled that urgently needed to get back on track. Mental health reform, one of my priorities when I was appointed minister in 2016, needed more attention to move that process along. There were several other projects to resume work on, but some of the pandemic-related pressure needed to be taken off me and off the team. I couldn't afford for them to continue to be blamed for the poor vaccine take-up and the inadequacies in the rollout. They, and seventeen thousand other people, had been working overtime for over a year to provide health services to a population that didn't seem to care enough about itself to take precautions against catching the virus. The decision was made to shift some responsibility for the rollout to another entity.

By mid-October, we finally started seeing signs that we were emerging from the third wave of COVID-19. Infections had gradually begun to fall after (as later identified) a peak on September 6. The series of lockdown days and nightly curfews may have had an impact on the number of new cases. Public health was concerned that though the infections were down, the decline in the positivity rate had slowed down, and the reproductive rate showed signs that it was trending up, and that we had not yet reached a safe place to remove the curfew. They were already looking ahead to December and keeping restrictions through the Christmas holiday. Nevertheless, by the end of October, Sundays were no longer designated as no-movement days, and by mid-November the curfew was moved to 9:00 pm, and gathering limits relaxed some more.

On Monday October 11, 2021, Cabinet officially resumed in-person meetings after approximately ten months of convening remotely. It was meant to be a signal to the country that things were to return to normal. We had to bring the country to the realization we had accepted: the goal of "zero COVID-19" was unachievable. The SARS-COV2 virus was here to stay. The idea was we would begin to treat COVID-19 as endemic, move out of pandemic mode and begin the transition to getting the country back to full productive capacity. We started the process of learning to live with COVID-19.

We continued to debate mandatory vaccination policies. Should we, or should we not? Jamaica was one of the countries with the lowest vaccine coverage in the world. There was, as with everything in this pandemic, pressure from both the "fors" and the "againsts." The PM, who had early on stated that mandatory vaccination might be against citizens' constitutional rights, was coming around to the idea that the laissez-faire approach we had been pursuing was not getting the country even near to where it needed to be for the vaccine to have a meaningful effect. News reports speculated that the PM was softening on his earlier position that vaccines would not be mandated. We were working with the idea that any mandatory vaccination policy we pursued would be to compel vaccination by direct or indirect threats of imposing restrictions in cases of non-compliance. But we were not agreed on what form it should take and if we would even call it a mandatory vaccination policy, given how contentious an issue it was. Other Caribbean countries were beginning to consider and implement them. Two Caribbean jurists gave a legal opinion that the constitution supported mandatory vaccines.

As we had all throughout the pandemic thus far, we took the WHO position into primary consideration: they did not support COVID-19 vaccination mandates or agree that COVID-19 vaccination should be a condition of international travel. From before September, several countries began disallowing unvaccinated non-nationals from crossing their borders, Canada being one, and the expectation was that the United States would soon follow, which it did.

There were many potential drawbacks. Where vaccine hesitancy was widely acknowledged to be rooted in lack of trust in government, forcing or trying to force people to take them would exacerbate that distrust and further harden it into resentment. Fake vaccination cards would almost certainly go into circulation, undermining trust and confidence in vaccinations cards in general.

But what were we to do? Though we didn't have comprehensive data, from what we could gather, fewer than 50 percent of nurses had been vaccinated, and some 30 percent of doctors working in the public sector had also not taken the vaccine. We couldn't force them to take it, and we couldn't afford to not let them work if they didn't take it. If we couldn't get the people on the frontline, the ones with medical knowledge, the ones most at risk, how could we expect to get the average, skeptical citizen to take it?

As we continued to deliberate on vaccine mandates, we sought to introduce new ways of getting more people vaccinated. Towards the end of October, house-to-house vaccination began in several parishes. Vaccines were taken to communities that were not close to a fixed site and to persons who were not able to travel to the sites. By this time also, around a hundred private doctors were certified to administer COVID-19 vaccines in their practices.

Vaccine supplies were adequate. We had received over two million vaccine doses. We had discarded 12 percent of them, which, while regrettable, was within the international best practice of 10 to 30 percent. The days of a national crisis over one missing vial of vaccine were a far distant memory. In mid-December, we launched digital vaccination cards and made provision for people to receive a third COVID-19 vaccine dose as a booster.

The virus continued to mutate. At the end of November 2021, the WHO declared the Omicron variant, first identified in Botswana, a variant of concern. A travel ban was imposed on South Africa and other southern African countries, though it was soon lifted, as it became clear that the variant was spreading rapidly across the world and would become the dominant variant everywhere.

It was unclear what the Omicron variant would mean for Jamaica. Would it bring a fourth wave? Nevertheless, from December 10, the curfew was extended another hour, to 10:00 pm, with 1:00 am curfews for Christmas Eve night and New Year's Eve night. Operating hours for beaches, rivers, and water attractions were extended from 4:00 pm to 5:00 pm. But by this point, it didn't seem that many people were obeying any of the restrictions, and enforcement was low. It was announced that the mandatory work-from-home order for the public sector would come to an end on December 31. The decision was taken for schools to reopen for in-person teaching in January, regardless of the vaccination rate of the students, and instructions were given to schools to start preparations for that.

For the first time since January 2020, I had a sense that we might be seeing the end of this pandemic.

Breach |

On March 15, 2022, almost two years to the day of the first case of COVID-19 in Jamaica, I breached the pandemic rules, and I was caught. I was photographed without a mask at a public event. The event was an album launch for one of Jamaica's most sensational artistes, Shenseea. I think she is incredibly talented, and I was very happy to be there seeing her perform and celebrating this achievement. She had also done some pro-vaccine messaging for the ministry, and so it was only right to show my support for her.

I wasn't the only enthusiastic fan. Several other senior government ministers also attended, and at least six of us where photographed enjoying ourselves, hugging, and taking selfies. Most of us were not wearing masks.

What was not known beyond a very small group of people then, however, and maybe up to now it is still not known, was that the previous day, cabinet had decided we would lift all COVID-19 restrictions, including mandatory mask wearing. It just had not been announced yet. It would be announced on March 17, two days later, to take effect on March 18. Inadvertently, I and my cabinet colleagues were celebrating early. We should not have. Further, it meant that my own personal record of making it through the pandemic without incident was marred.

That was another thing that I don't think many people appreciated: how many health ministers around the world had not made it through the pandemic without incident. While there were calls for my resignation during the pandemic, neither I nor anyone else took them seriously. I was fortunate to have a great deal of public support throughout my time as minister, including during the pandemic, as reflected in several opinion polls. And I didn't break any rules.

Others were not so fortunate. From the beginning, health officials got themselves into trouble. In early April 2020, Scotland's chief medical officer, Catherine Calderwood, resigned after she was found to have flouted her own advice on coronavirus by travelling to her second home. She was photographed by a tabloid newspaper at this property, more than an hour's drive from her home in Edinburgh.[77] The next month, the Bahamas health minister, Dr. Duane Sands, resigned after allowing six American citizens to disembark a plane along with a donation of COVID-19 test kits and swabs, five weeks after the March 27 border closure, while hundreds of Bahamians were stuck overseas waiting to go home. His reason was that he wanted to obtain the much-needed testing swabs.[78] Also in May, Brazil's health minister, Nelson Teich, resigned. He was at odds with President Jair Bolsonaro, who was urging Brazilians to defy lockdown orders from states and municipalities, at a time when Brazil had the second-highest death rate in the world.[79] This came one month after the president fired his predecessor, Luiz Henrique Mandetta, for imposing quarantine measures. In July, New Zealand's health minister resigned after he breached lockdown rules when he took his family to the beach.[80]

UK had its share of scandals. In June 2021, UK Health Secretary Matt Hancock, who had led the country's response to the coronavirus, resigned after being found to have breached social distancing rules with an aide with whom he was allegedly having an affair. Closed-circuit television images were taken of him and his paramour embracing and kissing. This was before lockdown rules were eased to allow hugs and

---

77 "Scotland's Chief Medical Officer Resigns After Flouting Coronavirus Lockdown Rules," Civil Service World, www.civilserviceworld.com/professions/article/scotlands-chief-medical-officer-resigns-after-flouting-coronavirus-lockdown-rules.
78 "Bahamas Health Minister Resigns After Breaching COVID-19 Protocol," *Caribbean National Weekly*, www.caribbeannationalweekly.com/caribbean-breaking-news-featured/bahamas-health-minister-resigns-after-breaching-covid-19-protocol/.
79 "Brazil Health Minister Nelson Teich Resigns After Clashes With Bolsonaro," *The New York Times*, www.nytimes.com/2020/05/15/world/americas/brazil-health-minister-bolsonaro.html.
80 "North Korea Declares Emergency in Border Town Over First Suspected COVID-19 Case," BBC News, www.bbc.com/news/world-asia-53259236.

other physical contact with people outside one's own household.[81] Incidentally, Neil Ferguson, the UK scientist who was instrumental in designing the nation's COVID-19 response, resigned for a similar reason much earlier in the pandemic. He had broken the lockdown order to meet with his married lover.[82] Then there was the scandal around the prime minister himself, who attended his own birthday party in the Cabinet Room at 10 Downing Street in the early days of the lockdown in May 2020. Though he was not made to resign (he was sanctioned), that event and the scandal surrounding it contributed to the weakening of his hold on his position, and he ultimately stepped down in 2022.[83]

Breaching lockdown rules was not the only infraction that forced people out of office. In August 2020, Poland's health minister, Łukasz Szumowski, unexpectedly announced his resignation just one day after his deputy minister, Janusz Cieszyński, had also resigned amid accusations that the health ministry had purchased defective masks from a friend of his family and overpriced respirators from a former arms dealer.[84] On a sad note, reminiscent of two incidents that happened in Jamaica, in January 2021, the Mongolian prime minister, Khurelsukh Ukhnaa, along with the entire cabinet, resigned after a mother and her newborn baby succumbed to COVID-19, allegedly due to apathy shown by health officials.[85]

---

81 "Europe Struggles as New COVID-19 Wave Gathers Pace," Associated Press, https://apnews.com/article/europe-coronavirus-pandemic-business-health-government-and-politics-eda28abad97e2ceb79f27abb71581421.

82 "Neil Ferguson Resigns After Breaking Lockdown to See Married Lover," Insider, www.insider.com/neil-ferguson-resigns-broke-lockdown-to-see-married-lover-2020-5.

83 "UK COVID-19: Boris Johnson Announces Plan B Measures," BBC News, www.bbc.com/news/uk-61137123.

84 "Unexpected Resignations of Polish Health Minister and Deputy Prompt Speculation and Concern," Notes from Poland, https://notesfrompoland.com/2020/08/19/unexpected-resignations-of-polish-health-minister-and-deputy-prompt-speculation-and-concern

85 "Mishandling of COVID Prompts Health Ministers of World to Quit," India Today, www.indiatoday.in/coronavirus-outbreak/story/mishandling-of-covid-prompts-health-ministers-of-world-to-quit-1809964-2021-06-02.

Once vaccines came into play, they also were the downfall of many. In February 2021, Peru's health minister, Dr. Pilar Mazzetti, resigned from her post after it was found that the former president of Peru Martin Vizcarra was vaccinated even before the vaccines were made available to the public.[86] That same month in Argentina, the health minister Gines Gonzalez Garcia submitted his resignation after irregularities appeared in the country's vaccination programme, and it was found that people have been using their clout to jump the queue.[87] The very next month in Ecuador, Health Minister Rodolfo Farfan resigned from his post three weeks after he was appointed. He was accused of favouritism in the country's vaccine rollout scheme and was being investigated for the same. Farfan had replaced Juan Carlos Zevallos, who resigned a month before, after allegedly participating in an inoculation effort at a nursing home where his mother lives.[88]

Then there were those who didn't make it because of politics and stress. In March 2021, the Slovakian health minister Marek KrajÃ resigned from his post when the ally parties in the coalition government alleged he failed in the handling of the pandemic, and over an alleged difference of opinion regarding the Russian Sputnik V vaccine.[89] The following month Austria's health minister Rudolf Anschober resigned, saying that he was "overworked" due to the COVID situation in the country and felt that the country needed a fitter person for the role. Anschober said that he was advised the same by his doctors.[90]

---

86 "Mishandling of COVID Prompts Health Ministers of World to Quit," *India Today*, www.indiatoday.in/coronavirus-outbreak/story/mishandling-of-covid-prompts-health-ministers-of-world-to-quit-1809964-2021-06-02.
87 "Mishandling of COVID Prompts Health Ministers of World to Quit," *India Today*, www.indiatoday.in/coronavirus-outbreak/story/mishandling-of-covid-prompts-health-ministers-of-world-to-quit-1809964-2021-06-02.
88 "Mishandling of COVID Prompts Health Ministers of World to Quit," *India Today*, www.indiatoday.in/coronavirus-outbreak/story/mishandling-of-covid-prompts-health-ministers-of-world-to-quit-1809964-2021-06-02.
89 "Mishandling of COVID Prompts Health Ministers of World to Quit," *India Today*, www.indiatoday.in/coronavirus-outbreak/story/mishandling-of-covid-prompts-health-ministers-of-world-to-quit-1809964-2021-06-02.
90 "Mishandling of COVID Prompts Health Ministers of World to Quit," *India Today*, www.indiatoday.in/coronavirus-outbreak/story/mishandling-of-covid-prompts-health-ministers-of-world-to-quit-1809964-2021-06-02.

The Czech Republic had four health ministers resign during the pandemic, for different reasons. Peter Arenberger resigned over irregularities in his tax returns. His predecessor, Jan Blatny, was fired for imposing strict conditions on the use of experimental drugs to treat COVID-19 patients and his refusal to accept Russia's Sputnik V vaccine, which had not been approved by the European Union's drug regulator. Blatny had replaced epidemiologist Roman Prymula, who was dismissed after he was photographed visiting a restaurant that should have been closed as part of the country's restrictive measures. Prymula, in turn, had replaced Adam Vojtech amid disagreement over the approach to managing the pandemic. Adam Vojtech was then reappointed to replace Arenberger.[91]

Relatively speaking then, I survived that long only to blunder right at the very end. I was roundly—and rightfully—criticized. I was lucky: when another cabinet member was videoed breaking COVID-19 restrictions by celebrating his advisor's birthday with several other people in a hotel bar, he was forced to resign as minister. I had better timing and didn't have to pay such a high price. The prime minister imposed fines on me and the other offenders. I wrote a cheque for J$100,000 to the Mustard Seed Foundation, one of Jamaica's most important charities.

---

91 "Europe Faces Tough Choices as COVID-19 Pandemic Continues," Associated Press, https://apnews.com/article/europe-pandemics-coronavirus-pandemic-health-government-and-politics-ac1a2f335b6676abb6bbe2ac0c530fc0.

We Made It |

That I was still health minister in March 2022 was remarkable, relative to the less salutary trajectories of so many of my counterparts across the world. In December 2021, there was talk of a cabinet reshuffle, and my name was the first to be called in the various discussions, publicly and, I'm certain, privately, about who would be moved and removed. This followed from the JLP's annual conference in November 2021, when I was not given an opportunity to speak. Because of the pandemic gathering restrictions, it was a "blended" conference, where fifty people were at the National Arena in Kingston, and five hundred delegates were in ten locations across the island where they were linked via live stream. I was on the arena stage, but the programme had it that I never got up from my seat. I found it peculiar but shrugged off overthinking it until I was approached by a senior member of the organization. That person argued that it "looked away" that at a party conference where the pandemic was the central point of the discussions, I, the front and point person for the pandemic response, was not given a platform to say even a word.

My conclusion was that my non-appearance at that critical juncture was an indication of the dissatisfaction with my holding the public health line in the pandemic management. From early on in the pandemic, I found myself in the middle of the debate between opening up and imposing restrictions. Perhaps this was the price to pay for being the standard bearer in this national public health crisis, where there were contending forces and interests.

I began to entertain thoughts such as, "Is this the time for me to begin decelerating my political career? Should I use this opportunity to remove myself entirely from the cabinet and become a backbencher for the first time in my political career? Would now be the time to put succession plans into action in my constituency?" By the second week of January 2022, however, the reshuffle was announced, and I was not among the ones shuffled.

In any case, I was focused on the fourth wave of COVID-19.

The Omicron variant spread like fire, raising new case numbers up to 1,400 and more a day. By this time, home testing kits were available, and we assumed many were not testing at all so that was likely an underestimate. Jamaica was one of many countries that experienced a surge in infections at the beginning of 2022, as the variant smashed infection records across Europe, North America, Africa, and Australia. Earlier in the pandemic, such a vertical rise in cases would have triggered stringent lockdowns.[92] But not this time. Instead, schools were reopening, and we were preparing Jamaica for "living with COVID-19." Though our vaccination rate was still abysmally low, and so we couldn't bank on that to protect people from severe illness, early indications were that Omicron was a gentler variant. It was far more contagious than previous variants, but far fewer people were dying. A 10:00 pm to 5:00 am curfew remained, but aside from that, mostly everything else moved towards normalization or, more accurately, the "new normal."

On March 17, 2022, during his contribution to the 2022/23 Budget Debate in the House of Representatives, the prime minister announced that all COVID-19 restrictions would be lifted when the Disaster Risk Management Act (DRMA) expired on March 18, at midnight. One month later, on April 16, 2022, COVID-19 travel restrictions were removed.

By May 3, 2022, when I gave my sectoral presentation, with the theme "Review, Reform, Renew," the main COVID-19 related work was dealing with the post-pandemic effects and efforts and activities related to that. Mental health, the surgery backlog, healthcare workers' fatigue and burnout, and a recognition programme were high on the agenda, and I was very deliberate in including those several other aspects of the ministry's work.

---

92 "Omicron Cases Are Exploding, Scientists Still Don't Know How Bad the Wave Will Be," *Science Magazine*, https://www.science.org/content/article/omicron-cases-are-exploding-scientists-still-don-t-know-how-bad-wave-will-be.

Here are excerpts from 2022 sectoral:

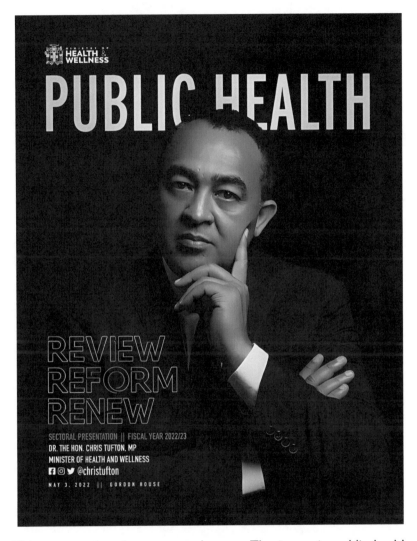

This was not just form over substance. The issues in public health that obtained before the pandemic still pertained. The NCDs crisis persisted, the need for investment in technology and infrastructure remained, and dengue was still an ongoing concern. The pandemic may have turned the world upside down and brought much of public health to a singular focus, but the pre-existing issues did not go away.

Front of Package Labeling

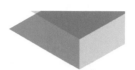

Madam Speaker, we will continue to reset our policies and laws to create a more health and wellness conscious citizen. The discussions around the consumers' right to know what is in their foods will continue this year with stepped up advocacy around finding a simple and consistent way to read labels and know the amount of salts, sugars and fats in our foods. Last year, Cabinet took a decision to support front of package labeling. This is a step in the right direction. This year we must decide on what this means and how it will be implemented. What is clear, Madam Speaker, is that we cannot have this kind of sick profile and

associated costs to the country and Jamaicans and not give our consumers at least a fair chance of making informed choices of the foods they eat. It is wrong - immoral and contrary to our international obligations to ensure the attainment of good health.

To manufacturers and food distributors I say, let us work together to improve the wellness and wellbeing of our consumers. It's a great way to build brand loyalty.

There are a number of significant areas of focus we will be pushing this year as part of the principle of Primordial Prevention.

684,900 Jamaicans have Hypertension

688,800 Jamaicans have Pre-hypertension

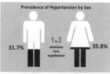

Prevalence of Hypertension by Sex

31.7%   1 in 3 Jamaicans have hypertension   35.8%

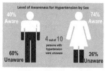

Level of Awareness for Hypertension by Sex

40% Aware   74% Aware

4 out of 10 persons with hypertension were unaware

60% Unaware   26% Unaware

Classification of Adults According to BMI

Nutritional status	BMI (kg/m²)
Underweight	Below 18.5
Normal weight	18.5–24.9
Overweight (BMI ≥25 kg/m²)	
Pre-obesity	25.0–29.9
Obesity class I	30.0–34.9
Obesity class II	35.0–39.9
Obesity class III	Above 40

Source: WHO (2000) Obesity: preventing and managing the global epidemic. Report of a WHO Consultation (WHO Technical Report Series 894)

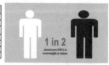

Trends among persons 15-74 years for 2001, 2008, 2017

Condition	2001 (%)	2008 (%)	2017 (%)	% Change
Overweight (BMI ≥ 25)	45.7	51.8	53.9	17.9
Obesity (BMI ≥ 30)	19.7	25.3	28.9	46.7
Hypertension	20.9	25.2	31.5	50.7
Diabetes mellitus	7.2	7.9	10.2	41.7
High Cholesterol	14.6	11.7	17.1	17.1

1 in 2 Jamaicans (50%) is overweight or obese

577,300 Jamaicans are Obese

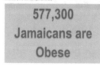

Distribution of Nutritional Status (%) by Sex

P<0.001 for male: female difference in weight distribution

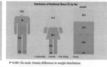

Trends among persons 15-74 years for 2001, 2008, 2017

Condition	2001 (%)	2008 (%)	2017 (%)	% Change
Overweight (BMI ≥ 25)	45.7	51.8	53.9	17.9
Obesity (BMI ≥ 30)	19.7	25.3	28.9	46.7
Hypertension	20.9	25.2	31.5	50.7
Diabetes mellitus	7.2	7.9	10.2	41.7
High Cholesterol	14.6	11.7	17.1	17.1

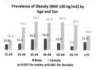

Prevalence of Obesity (BMI ≥30 kg/m2) by Age and Sex

Male   Female
p=0.037 for males; p<0.001 for females

The cabinet ministers' contribution to the sectoral debates are usually a special occasion. The minister's leadership team, key constituents, and close family and friends usually attend and sit in the visitors' gallery at Gordon House, where Parliament meets. In 2020, four people attended my presentation, as at that time no one was allowed to attend Parliament in the gallery. In 2021, there were just over two dozen, as gathering rules meant that numbers were limited and there had to be empty seats in between each attendee. In 2022, the gallery was full to capacity. That was as clear a sign as any that the pandemic was behind us.

And yet, was it?

Postscript |

After three years of COVID-19 being a central theme in my sectoral presentation, on May 3, 2023, it was a mere paragraph. I noted that while the pandemic was well over and done with, people were still contracting the virus and had died since the beginning of the year. By then, one might spot someone wearing a mask here and there, but it was far from the norm. The ministry's chief epidemiologist was one of the few, and she was extremely disciplined about it. I still hadn't contracted the virus, as far as I knew.

Two days after the presentation, on May 5, 2023, the WHO announced that COVID-19 no longer qualified as a global emergency. Though almost every country in the world had long since "returned to normal" by then, it was worth marking as a symbolic end to the pandemic. With that, I considered the worst health catastrophe the world experienced in a century to have closed its final chapter.

Acknowledgements |

I am deeply grateful to the Most Honourable Prime Minister, the cabinet, and to the following individuals and groups whose unwavering support and dedication have been instrumental in Jamaica's journey through the COVID-19 pandemic:

Permanent Secretary Dunstan Bryan, for his tireless commitment to navigating the complexities of our healthcare system during those challenging times.

Chief Medical Officer Jacqueline Bisasor-McKenzie, whose expertise and leadership were invaluable in guiding our public health response.

Chief Epidemiologist Dr. Karen Webster-Kerr, for her invaluable contributions to our understanding of the epidemiological landscape and for guiding our strategies accordingly.

I am indebted to the prime minister of Jamaica, Hon. Andrew Holness, and the cabinet for entrusting me with the responsibility to provide the necessary leadership in that critical moment in our nation's history.

To Jamaica's private sector leaders who provided invaluable advice and critical support, often in the face of difficult decisions that were both unusual and unpopular, I offer my sincere appreciation.

I extend my heartfelt gratitude to the thousands of public health workers who have selflessly sacrificed themselves to safeguard the health and well-being of our fellow Jamaicans. Their courage and dedication inspire us all.

Last but by no means least, I would like to express a special thanks to Dr. Diana Thorburn, whose guidance and editorial judgement made this manuscript possible.

About Chris Tufton |

Chris Tufton is a Jamaican public figure and writer who has navigated a trajectory that transcends conventional roles in academia, business, public policy research, and national politics. His debut book, *State of Mind: Politics, Uncertainty, and the Search for the Jamaican Dream* (Ian Randle Press, 2019), intricately weaves a narrative of resilience and political awakening, culminating in his re-election to Parliament in 2016.

Armed with a doctorate in business administration (DBA), Chris Tufton, an alumnus of renowned institutions like Manchester High School, the University of the West Indies at Mona (Jamaica), Georgia State University (USA), and the University of Manchester (UK), has been a member of Jamaica's Parliament between 2007 and 2011, and again from 2016 to the date of writing. His influence in crisis management and health policies reflects a multifaceted approach to public service, making him a national leader of distinction.

In this second book, *Wild Flavours: An Insider's Account of Jamaica's Journey through the Crisis of the COVID-19 Pandemic*, Tufton unfolds an unprecedented behind-the-scenes chronicle of his tenure as Jamaica's minister of health and wellness during the COVID-19 pandemic. The book offers profound insights into crisis leadership, communication, team building, community mobilization, and multilateral cooperation— essential components in overcoming this existential threat.

Wild Flavours transcends the boundaries of a mere pandemic chronicle. It's an exploration of crisis leadership in action, guided by Tufton's authoritative voice and shaped by his pivotal role as portfolio minister. The book stands as a testament to Tufton's commitment to public service, spotlighting his calming maturity and judgment crucial for overcoming fears, uncertainties, and coordinating stakeholders through anxieties, distress, and outright resistance during the pandemic.

This book is a must-read for those seeking an insider's perspective on leading in crisis situations and should be prescribed reading for students of public health leadership.

Made in the USA
Columbia, SC
11 October 2024

43434236R10174